Now that I have cancer . . . I am whole

Rev. Steve & Jackie Bard
17314 Lee Ln.
Harlan, IN 46743

NOW THAT I HAVE CANCER . . . I AM WHOLE

JOHN ROBERT McFARLAND

John Robert McFarland (signature)

Meditations for cancer patients and those who love them

NIGHT SONG PRESS
1-888-648-7664
425 20th Place S.W.
Mason City, IA 50401

Now that I Have Cancer . . .
I Am Whole
© 1993 John Robert McFarland
For information write
Andrews and McMeel,
a Universal Press Syndicate Company,
4900 Main Street,
Kansas City, Missouri 64112.

Design by Cameron Poulter

Library of Congress Cataloging-in-Publication Data

McFarland, John Robert.
    Now that I have cancer—I am whole : meditations for cancer
patients and those who love them / John Robert McFarland.
      p.   cm.
    ISBN 0-8362-2424-8 : $14.95. — ISBN 0-8362-2426-4 (pbk.) : $8.95
    1. McFarland, John Robert. 2. Cancer—Patients—Religious life.
3. Cancer—Patients—Biography. 4. Cancer—Religious aspects—
Christianity. I. Title.
BV4910.33.M34   1993
242'.4—dc20   93-31928
                                                                 CIP

This is for my wife, Helen Karr McFarland,
and for our daughters,
Mary Beth and Kathleen Anne.

Without you, I would not be alive.
Without you, I would never have been alive.

Contents

CONTENTS

CONTENTS

CONTENTS

Acknowledgments

I WANT TO THANK all the good folks at the Carle Cancer Center in Champaign, Illinois—especially my oncologist, Alan Hatfield, his nurse practitioner, Marie Deschamps, and all my nurses, the pharmacists, the social workers, and the front desk personnel. Becky, Evelyn, Sarah, Olivia, Barry, Toni, Judy, Linda, Joni, Laura, Melissa, Nancy, Ron, Joan, Jill, Sharon, Pam, Debbi—I hope you know how important you are to those of us who love you so much but never want to see you again! My sincere appreciation goes as well to my family physician, Robert Arrol, and his staff, and to the surgical and nursing staffs at Covenant Hospital in Urbana, Illinois.

Special thanks go to all the members of the Carle cancer support group, and our social worker and friend, Jeanette Pritschet. I've not only been supported by them, but I've learned so much from them.

There couldn't have been a better group to learn from than my classmates in "Empowering the Cancer Patient" at Iliff Seminary in Denver, in the summer of 1990. John Anduri, Paul Hamilton, M.D., and Lynn Ringer, the leaders of that group, have made wholeness in the midst of cancer possible not only for Helen and me, but for literally thousands of other cancer patients. Their story is told in *I'm a Patient, Too*, by Albert Hill.

Various of these meditations were read by fellow patients Jean Cramer-Heuerman, Nancy Nichols, and Kim Wagler, while the thoughts were still in the hatching stage, and I thank them for their kindness.

Kim Wagler was my first cancer nurse. Hardly a year had gone by after she initiated me into the mysteries of chemotherapy and how to deal with it than she became a cancer patient, too. She is precious to me not only as my nurse but as a fellow traveler in the cancer journey.

Rose Mary Shepherd and Rachael Grace Richardson have been guides and models in the cancer walk. Sharon Butts has walked it with me, even though she's never had it. Thank you.

Through the dedication, my debt to my wife and daughters is made clear. As well, I have been formed by a large, extended family of Ponds and McFarlands that always gave me a sense of belonging. My parents, John F. and Mildred Pond McFarland, my brother, Jim, and my sisters, Mary V. Lindquist and Margaret Ann Vermond, are more dear to me than they will ever know.

I have been supported through my cancer time by more people in more churches than I can possibly name. Especially important to me, however, are those of the Forsythe United Methodist Church, near Oakland City, Indiana, and those of Arcola, Illinois. The good folk of Forsythe accepted me and loved me as a child and teenager. The family of the Arcola United Methodist Church kept me going through the difficult days of recovery from surgery and chemotherapy. Moreover, they let me minister to them by getting well in front of them. For that, I'll be forever grateful.

And BUMBS, you know who you are, you know how much you mean to me.

Early in the publishing process, I asked a suspicious question of Donna Martin, the Vice President and Editorial Director of Andrews and McMeel. She said, "Don't worry. I think you'll find that we're nice people." Truer words were never spoken! In addition to Donna herself, they include especially Patty Donnelly, Dorothy O'Brien, Jean Lowe, Kathy Viele, and Matt Lombardi. They also include Anne Gaudinier, Rick Harris, and Rich Romaniano of HarperAudio. And isn't that a beautiful cover that George Diggs designed?

The poem "Endangered Species" originally appeared in the April 1991 edition of *The Midwest Poetry Review*.

"Stealing Donkeys" appeared in a somewhat different form in *The Christian Century* of March 28, 1990. The poem "Pain" appeared in the same publication for November 14, 1990.

Introduction

I NEVER EXPECTED TO GET CANCER. Before me, there had been only two cases of cancer among the several hundred relatives who inhabit four generations of McFarlands and Ponds. Both of those were well past their eightieth birthday at the first sign.

I had lived a healthy lifestyle. I was a long-distance runner and a third baseman. I'd received a lot of satisfaction from my work and a lot of love from my family and friends.

I had no symptoms of any kind, until a midnight pain "down south" caused the surgeon to have a look. He ended up cutting out a third of my colon and a malignant tumor.

An oncologist came to my room and announced, "You've got it." I had no idea what "it" was. Cancer had never occurred to me, not even as I went to surgery. The oncologist said I had a 70 percent chance of recurrence in one to two years and that there was no adjuvant therapy that would do me any good. I heard that as a death sentence; I would be dead in one to two years.

I was thrown for a loop. My life was turned totally upside down. The change was so complete that I started every sentence with "Now that I have cancer . . . ," a phrase that marked off my present days from all that had been before. My friend Bill White, who appears in the "Touching Time" meditation, must have gotten tired of hearing it, because he said, "That sounds like the title of a book." So it is.

It started as a cancer journal. Keeping a journal came naturally to me; I like to write things down and I like to keep records. Also, however, I read that the recovery rate

for cancer patients who put down their thoughts and feelings in a journal is much better than for those who don't. I
wasn't about to pass up an opportunity like that!

As I wrote I realized that I wasn't just in a journal, I was
on a journey, although I wasn't sure of the destination. I
came to understand that many others are on that same
journey, with similar doubts about where it will lead and
where it will end. I became less and less satisfied with simply recording my own expedition. I knew I needed to say a
word to and for the others who share the cancer walk.
These are my meditations, but they are not mine alone. I
like to think of this as a common journal for all of us who
must make this trip.

So this book is in part the story of my own cancer journey and those who support me in it. It is also the story of
the journeys of others, who have honored me by letting me
walk a way with them and learn from them. Most importantly, it is a way of sharing the journey. We know "you've
got to walk that lonesome valley by yourself." We also
know, paradoxically, that we need company on that trip.
We're alone and yet together, what a friend of mine once
called "a sense of shared privacy."

I have written each meditation from my own experience
rather than in generalized fashion, because cancer is a very
individual disease. We are not statistics or percentages or
categories; we are persons. Cancer is, however, an equal-
opportunity disease. It strikes rich and poor, young and old,
good and bad, "red and yellow, black and white." In that
way we all share the same road. I trust that in these meditations you will see your own story as I share mine.

We are on a journey, but it is a trip of individual steps.
We need to live in the moment, and sometimes that's all we

can do. We get by one day at a time, and often only one minute at a time. It's sometimes difficult for us even to hold a big book, yet alone read one. We concentrate best in short bursts, on one idea at a time. It is hard to sort through many pages and long chapters, raw knowledge and strange new terms, to find the words we need to hear in our particular moment of need.

So this book is divided into categories that we cancer patients understand—steps of the journey. There is no "beginning" and no "end." Feel free to read the meditations in whatever order is best for you, according to which step you're taking at the moment.

The life change that cancer forces is so huge, so overwhelming, especially if surgery or chemotherapy or radiation adds another misery to the mix. It's hard to get hold of, like trying to play catch with a watermelon when you've been used to a baseball. So we tend to pick up on the little changes and events of cancer. It's easier to talk about "making offerings to the big white god" or how we'll look in a wig than to consider whether chemo will actually move us toward a cure.

That's good. We live in stories, not in abstract theories. Dealing with strange bras and stuck eyelids and bald heads will lead us on to the wider and deeper issues easily enough. The little changes break open the potential for meaning, like the little change in an eggshell at a chick's first peck. So these meditations usually start with some mundane observation or event, like getting sick when I see Becky, my chemo pusher, even if I see her at a theater. They start there because those are the events of our cancer journey. What they mean . . . well, we can consider that as we walk along together.

It was on my birthday that they cut me open and found the cancer. It was on Helen's birthday that I began a year of chemotherapy. My veins started breaking down from the chemo, so I had to get a Groshong catheter in my chest to save the veins. They installed that on our wedding anniversary, of course. We began to dread special days! We came to understand, though, that even with—and perhaps especially with—cancer, every day is a special day.

It was on those special days that I wrote these meditations, and I have left them as they were then—when I first heard "that word," when the chemotherapy made me "call Ralph on the big white phone," when I wondered what I'd done to cause this, when I was sick and tired of being sick and tired.

I'm through with chemo now, feeling good, getting a little anxious as test time approaches. There's a temptation to go back and rewrite the meditations of the early days and the chemo days and the down days, to give them the benefit of the long view. I've not yielded to that temptation, though. At each of those steps, the way it is is the way it is. When you're there, you're there. That's okay.

WHEN
YOU FIRST
HEAR
"THAT WORD"

. . . *I say "that word" all the time.*

CANCER! There. I did it.

Some folks are actually afraid of the word itself, aren't they? Have you noticed? They refer to your "trouble," or your "disease," or your "struggle." They just can't bring themselves to say CANCER.

I understand how they feel. I'm more than a little bit afraid of CANCER myself. That's why I say it every time I get the chance. CANCER.

People are afraid to speak that word because they know that words have power. Tell a child often enough that he's stupid, and he'll believe it. Tell her that she's bright, and she'll believe that, too.

A friend once asked me why our children "turned out so well." I can't understand why he seemed surprised that my kids weren't odd. I told him that it was simple: we just gave them everything they wanted and bragged on them all the time. (Our children tell a somewhat different version.) I firmly believe there will be enough people in life who will cut your children down that they don't need it from their parents, too. Brag on them; those words have power.

I know of a church on a university campus that was having trouble keeping its grass alive. The students were cutting across the churchyard on their way to classes and wearing a huge path in it. They put up a sign that said "Keep off the grass." It did no good at all. Then, however, they changed the sign to "Let it live." The students used the sidewalk. The right word is a lever that can move the world.

When I was little, my mother taught me a little epigram

2

to use against the neighborhood bullies: "Sticks and stones may break my bones, but words will never hurt me." It would have worked better if the bullies hadn't used sticks and stones as well as words! They certainly knew how to use words, though, and those hurt more than the sticks and stones. It's infuriating to be called "yellow" by three boys who are twice as big as you are. You know they are the true cowards, since they have to gang together and pick on someone smaller. As a child, however, you can't even find the right words so you can tell them that. You just run away.

Bob Simon, the CBS news reporter, was a prisoner of the Iraqis for several weeks during the Persian Gulf War. He said that the words were worse than the beatings. "After a while," he said, "you realize that a beating, although unpleasant and painful, will come to a stop. The terror they put into you with words, however, goes on and on."

Sticks and stones can break your bones, but the words of terror break your spirit.

The terror of that word, CANCER, can go on and on if we don't say it. Saying it puts it into the light and takes away so much of its power.

Sure, I'm still afraid. I could say CANCER all day long, and I'd keep on being scared. CANCER, though, when you speak it right out loud, isn't very strong. It has strength only in the dark. It can break my body. There may even be times when it will break my spirit. But I know that CANCER is weak. It can't break LOVE. There's no way CANCER can take me away from the love of my wife and my children and my family and my friends . . . and God.

> *Now that I have cancer, I say that word all the time.*
> *You know the one I mean—LOVE.*

. . . *Cancer is the answer.*

THAT'S WHAT A FRIEND TOLD ME when she first heard that word. "I've been looking for something all my life. I've tried booze and drugs and whatever else I could think of. I've been depressed for forty years. I prayed to die. Now, cancer is the answer."

I think I know what she meant. As I sat in my hospital bed, invaded by tubes and lost in a cloud of uncertainty, I had that same feeling. Oh, that wasn't all I felt. Anger and fear and despair and lostness and sadness and hope all called for their turn, too. But cancer was an answer. It pulled all the loose threads together. It was the pivot around which everything else whirled, like the post for a game of tetherball. No one, including me, looked for me to deal with anything else at all. That was a feeling of great relief. I could let loose of everything else, as a snake wiggles out of an old skin. It was all so simple—just cancer and me.

An oncologist's careless words helped that feeling along. I understood from him that I would be dead in a year or two. I would have thought it even had he not spoken the words. In our society, we equate cancer with death. Nothing focuses the mind like a literal deadline. I didn't like what I heard, but there were no distractions to it. Cancer was the answer; all my other concerns and worries were pushed aside, like so many unread newspapers that get tossed into the recycling bin while you're not looking. The deck is cleared.

Unlike my friend, I've rarely been depressed, but I was then. Studies show that a patient's condition deteriorates

4

rapidly right after hearing the diagnosis. Depression follows "that word" as surely as "Wait till next year" follows a Cubs fan. Depression is literally a low place. I wanted to sink down into that low place and stay there.

There's a seductiveness in cancer. It cleared my calendar so nicely. I could get ready to die with a clear conscience— nothing left undone since I couldn't be expected to do anything. It was the perfect excuse for not having to deal with anything. There's a perverse comfort in illness. You just lie there, no expectations.

While I was still in the hospital, recovering from surgery, a friend gave me a copy of Bernie Siegel's *Love, Medicine, and Miracles*. In it he asks, "Why do you need the cancer?" In other words, to what is it the answer? My friend says she needs it in order to die, the answer to her prayer. I guess my answer is that I needed to have my life simplified to the point that I got permission to concentrate on the only important thing there is.

Cancer is a very personal disease. We must each answer that question, "Why do you need it?" When we've answered, however, we find it's only the first question in a line that stretches clear over the hill. So I needed it to die, or to get clear of life's baggage, or something else. But what now? How do I deal with it? Do I just curl up and write "The End" to my story? Do I fight it somehow? It's just me and cancer, yes, eyeball to eyeball, like a matador and a bull in the middle of the ring, not even aware of the sun and the dust and the shouts of the crowd. But we still have to deal with each other. Who will blink first?

Cancer is the answer, but it's another question. What's important to me? What's the meaning of life? How do I find love?

We've looked for love, like my friend, in all the wrong places—in booze and dollars and degrees and promotions and sex and power and work and thrills. We've filled our lives with doing. So often our deeds have erased our actual lives, our being. The question now is not "What do I do?" but "Who am I?" We answer cancer not with more activities, although learning and treatment and meditation and visualization may be things we need to do.

We answer cancer with love, with simple being, with the knowledge that each life ends as it started—unbidden, naked, without knowledge of what will be. I am. I am, now, in this moment. There is no certainty in this life, only trust.

That's what I tried to say to my friend. Yes, cancer is the answer. You needed it, so you could be broken into pieces so small that you can be put back together in ways you've never even thought about. None of us needs death or cancer. They're just ways of telling us that we need love.

When Moses asked God for a name, God simply replied, "I am who I am." That's all there is. It comes to us at sunrise and sunset, in the simple act of kindness, in gentle human touch, in music that reaches the spirit deep within, in the knowledge that all that ever was and all that ever will be is here, right now, in this moment. We live by grace, not only in general, but moment to moment. Cancer tells me that.

Now that I have cancer, cancer is the answer.

WHEN
A PART
OF YOU
IS GONE

. . . A part of me is gone.

THEY TOOK OUT ONE THIRD OF MY COLON. I've "lost" it. I'm not "whole" anymore.

A lot of us are no longer "whole." Cancer patients lose breasts and kidneys and thyroids and lungs and sections of livers and about any other body part we can name. In treatment we can also lose hair and bowel control and even our dinner! We're not only unwhole, we're "losers," too.

Think about those common words—words like *whole* and *loser*. They take on different meanings when we put them in the cancer context, don't they?

Most of the time we can disguise the fact that we aren't whole, that we are losers. We have wigs and turbans and prostheses and body-hugging colostomy bags. They're good things. If you lose your teeth, you get false ones. What's wrong with doing the same thing if you lose breasts or hair? Sure, some of it's just "cosmetic," but there's nothing wrong with looking good. Anything we can do to feel better about ourselves, let's do it!

We know, however, even when we're looking our best, that there's something missing. Some losses can't be replaced. I'll never get another colon.

Jesus had something to say about this. "If your eye or your hand causes you to sin, pluck it out or cut it off and throw it away; it is better that you lose one of your members than that your whole body be thrown into hell. And if your hand causes you to sin, cut it off and throw it away" (Matthew 5:29–30).

8

(It's very easy to get lost in the trees here and thus not see the forest. Are heaven and hell literal places? Did Jesus mean you should physically cut off your hand? Interesting questions, but they are trees, not the forest.)

Sin breaks relationship. Sin breaks us apart from God and our neighbors and our own true selves. Sin fragments us, makes us "unwhole." Sin causes us to "lose" what is most important in life, the relationships through which love comes.

Ah, there are those words again—*unwhole, loser*.

Jesus is saying that it's not the physical loss that makes us unwhole, that makes us losers. In fact, he says, even if something so physically important as an eye or hand makes us lose that which is most important, love, then it is good to be a loser, good to be unwhole in our physical bodies so that we can be whole in love.

The point Jesus was making (the forest rather than the trees), is that true wholeness has nothing to do with whether our bodies would make good charts for anatomy students. The one who plucks out an eye or cuts off a hand because it is breaking relationships, because it is walling us off from love, is more whole than the one who's never lost a part but uses those parts to hurt.

I have a friend who always says, as he prays in church, "Bless those of us assembled here." It's a marvelous phrase. He means, of course, bless those of us who have come together in this one location from our separate places. The word "assembled" has an individual meaning, as well. It refers to each one of us being put together, being made whole. "Bless those of us who are being put together here."

Sin separates us. Coming together in love assembles us, puts us together.

9

In a strange way, I feel more assembled, more put to-gether, since I've lost a part of my body than I did before. Cancer has brought me closer to God and to those who love me and to my own true self. In that sense, good health was a sin. As long as I could keep going day by day without even thinking about my health, it was also easy for me to take love for granted. Like Scarlett O'Hara, I could think about that tomorrow.

Cancer reminds us that there is no tomorrow, just as there is no yesterday. For love, there is only today.

Now that I have cancer, a part of me is missing. Ironically, I'm more "whole," more a "winner," of love, than I've ever been before.

. . . I am learning to see myself through the eyes of love.

THOSE WHO LOVE ME have much better eyes than I. The eyes of love are always best. Love is not blind at all. Love sees with the eyes of God, not the eyes of the world. Love has remarkable clarity of vision, the scope of an eagle, free from all those floating debris spots of "reality."

There was something about me, before cancer, that I could not love. Not all of me, but something. I must have hated it so much, to create a cancer that required my own mutilation, to demand that a part of me be cut out and thrown away. I don't quite understand that, but somehow I feel its truth. It's like when you have set the alarm for six in the morning, and you wake up just before the bell rings for you, even though you normally snooze steadily on until seven. The body knows.

You may not feel that way at all. I have a cancer friend who says, "I'm blameless. I didn't do anything at all to cause this." I believe her. She knows herself. I know myself, too.

I look at me with the eyes of reality and what do I see? A scrawny, hairless man. Those formerly marvelous, marathoning muscles just hang on bones of unproductive and depleted marrow. The bright blue eyes are bloodshot. They peek out through tiny slits where my eyelids have glued themselves to each other. This skinny man is bent over, divided by an angry, red scar that looks like an N-gauge model railroad track. The veins beneath my skin look like jagged and jaded lightning flashes, as if I had gotten caught in a bleach storm in my Captain Marvel suit. My lips are red and puffy, like a sad circus clown. That's the view through the eyes of reality.

Then there are the eyes of love. My wife sighs, "Every time I look at you, I fall in love all over again." My daughters say, "Remember what good times we had when we were little girls and you lay down on the sofa after supper and we'd sit on the back of it and roll you off with our feet? You're the best dad ever." My teammates call to say, "Hurry back. Nobody else has the reflexes to play third base as close to the batter as you do." A woman tells me, "I'd be dead except for the hope you gave me." A now-grown man says, "You have no idea how important you were to all of us on campus in the sixties. You made us believe we could make a difference." God says, "I love you just the way you are."

Those aren't the eyes of reality; those are the eyes of love. They see me as I want to be and yet, for them, already am.

Now that I have cancer, I can see myself through their eyes. I like seeing me through the eyes of love.

. . . I sing.

I ALWAYS ENJOYED SINGING, but now I sing all the
time. It's almost impossible to sing a full-throated note
and be tied up by fear at the same time.

I sing all sorts of songs—hymns and ballads and pop and
scat and blues and rock and folk and opera—anything that
comes to mind. I make up crazy songs as I go along, too.
Sometimes the words make sense, sometimes not. Sometimes they rhyme, other times not. Some have familiar tunes,
but some of those I make up as well.

One of the most frustrating things for me when I first
came home from the hospital was that I couldn't sing. The
tube up my nose and down my throat left me sounding like
Donald Duck with a cold. I had been cut open from Los
Angeles to Boston. Every muscle in my abdomen was
spending all its energy just trying to get reconnected. I had
no power from my diaphragm. All I could do was mouth
the words.

Well, I decided, if that's all I can do, that's what I'll do.
Better to sing a wee, tiny song than no song at all.

Like most doors that close, this one caused another to
open. Since I couldn't sing very well, I began to compose.
"Compose" isn't quite the right word. I began to "adjust"
songs.

I sing them in the bathtub mostly. That's probably safest.
While I lie in the warm water, Emmett Kelly, the clown,
comes and sweeps my body clean, with his spotlight broom.
(If you've not read the meditation on commitment yet, see
page 44 for more about Emmett.) He does each part, each

13

organ, of my body. I sing to help him along. My, how that clown can sweep out cancer cells when he has a little music!

As I wash my hair, I sing "Gonna wash that cancer right out of my self . . . and send it on its way." I adjusted the spiritual "Oh, Freedom." I sing, "No more cancer. No more cancer. No more cancer inside of me. And before I'll be a slave, I'll put cancer in its grave, and go home to my Lord, and be free." How's about (to the tune of "If You're Happy and You Know It, Clap Your Hands"), "I'm glad I'm a little cake of soap. (Repeat.) I'll slippie and I'll slidie all over my hidie and I'll wash the cancer off with my soap."

Okay, so they're pretty bad, but they're just for Emmett and me, and they work.

I don't mean singing works by automatically wafting cancer away on a tune. It might help, but who knows? I do know that it works by taking away the fear.

You just can't sing and be afraid at the same time. That's why we sing in the dark. It is also very difficult to sing and "awfulize" at the same time. Awfulizing is the process of imagining all the awful things that might happen to us. We spend more time at it than we realize. The less awfulizing we do, the more likely we are to get well. The immune system doesn't like awfulizing; it does like singing.

Singing is as natural as loving. In fact, they are very closely related—two limbs from one trunk, from one root system. Together they spread out a canopy of shade.

Both those limbs get weather-beaten, however. They are besieged by frost and drought and hail and acid rain and parasites and blight. It's a wonder they survive at all, and in some folks I guess they don't. But their tree is rooted deep in the soil of the Spirit.

With all those blights and plights attacking them,

though, what was so natural becomes unnatural. How many people refuse to sing, claim they can't sing, give all sorts of excuses—from illness to shyness—why they mustn't sing. We do the same with loving. We're afraid we'll be hurt. We have already been hurt. We're afraid we'll be rejected or look silly.

I suspect we can learn a lot about how we love by how we sing.

The search for healing and wholeness includes singing. You don't have to go on stage. You don't even have to use a recognizable tune or sing on key. Just croak out whatever words you remember or that come to you. Sing your prayers and sing away your fears. Do it in the bathroom with the water running. Sing along with Johnny Mathis or Dolly Parton or Mick Jagger.

Singing leaves no room for fear. Even if singing doesn't cure us, it does help to heal us. That, after all, is the goal of life; not just to live a long time, but to live well.

> *Now that I have cancer, I sing. Try it . . .*
> *"Happy days are here again. The cancer's*
> *gone away again . . ."*

. . . *I do something each day.*

IT MAY NOT SOUND LIKE MUCH OF A GOAL, but three weeks after my surgery, "something every day" is a big step forward. Of course, I've been doing the necessities for recovering from surgery and to prevent complications—deep breathing, walking the loop from my bedroom to the family room and through the living room and back down the hall again, sleeping ten hours a night plus an afternoon nap, eating a gentle four meals a day. After all those necessaries are done, and I've read a few pages of Bernie Siegel or Greg Anderson or Joan Borysenko, "something" is all I have time and energy for.

By "something," I mean making a telephone call, or writing a letter, or doing the dishes. It's not much, is it? I used to run five miles and then work ten or twelve hours without a break. I made a dozen telephone calls and wrote enough letters to make the postal service smile and saw a mob of people, and still got the dishes done and walked the dog. Now Waggs just hangs around the door with drooping tail until Helen notices that it's walk time.

My daily "something" now, however, takes more concentration and planning and discipline than all the many tasks that used to race through my days, put together. I know that if I choose to write one letter, it means I can't write to anyone else. Which letter is most important? Or should I be sure today that Helen finds a clean kitchen when she returns home from a day of dealing with boisterous teenagers? When you have only one thing you can do, how do you decide which one thing it is?

Clear back in the summer of '64, when Henry Aaron was playing for the Braves and John Roseboro was catching for the Dodgers, Aaron came to bat in a game between the two teams. Roseboro noticed that Aaron had the brand of the bat to the front, toward the pitcher. The brand is the place where the information about the bat—the name of the manufacturer, etc.—is burned into the wood. Every sandlot baseball player knows you always bat with the brand to the back, because the bat is likely to break if it and the ball connect directly on the brand.

"Hey, you've got the brand to the front," said Roseboro.

Aaron looked at it, left it where it was, took his stance, and said, "I didn't come up here to read."

It's no surprise that Hank Aaron is the all-time leading home run hitter. He knew what his one "something" was; he was up there to hit.

It's important to concentrate on the one "something" I have to do, to experience it rather than just do it, to concentrate on it and feel it, rather than just marking it off a list so I can go on to something else.

As I come to bat, it's tempting to say the one thing I'm up here for is to get well, to hit the long ball, to take cancer over the wall and out of the park. I'd like that. The homer, though, is simply the end product of many little "somethings"—the openness of the stance, the tilt of the bat, the keenness of eye to see whether the pitch is in the strike zone, the shift of the weight, the snap of the wrists. All those little "somethings" put together were what made Aaron the homer champ.

My turn at bat isn't just to get well, but to do well, to concentrate on each event of the day, to pay attention to the little things, because the only way I have to love is in that one swing. My "something" each day now is more important than all the masses of things I used to do. Whether I live long or short, in pain or without pain, I have one thing to do each day, regardless of how many ways that one thing may be expressed. Into each letter, each phone call, each washed dish, I put the full measure of all my love. I think by doing well, I'm helping myself get well, but that's not the point. Søren Kierkegaard wrote that "purity of heart is to will one thing." Whether it's a home run or a sacrifice bunt, my turn at bat is to do one thing, to love.

Now that I have cancer, I do something each day.

. . . I'm learning to live with limits.

NOT THAT I DIDN'T HAVE LIMITS BEFORE. Before,
though, my limits were pretty far out. I knew I'd never
play first base for the Reds, or run a marathon under
three hours, or be asked to a dinner party at Sophia Loren's
house. But I could play third base for "The Fossils" in the
Rocking Chair League. I could run a marathon under four
hours. I was asked to dinner parties at Pat Meyerholtz's
house. Maybe I'll play softball with the old guys again
sometime. Maybe I'll even run a marathon again, when the
chemo is over and the Groshong catheter is out of my chest
and I'm not tired so much of the time. Pat and Roy still in-
vite me to their house, as do other friends. When the cold and
flu season is over and my immune system is no longer depressed, maybe I'll be able to enjoy those homemade rolls
and that home-style friendship once more.

In the meantime, I can't go to ball games, or restaurants,
or other places where people and germs gather. I can't do
anything where I'll get cut, because the Coumadin has
thinned my blood and I won't heal very well. Helen has to
crawl under the house to adjust the vents as the seasons
change. John Mills cleans my gutters. Bill Alexander mows
my yard. Ross and Paulina Hunt weed my flowers. Sometimes I feel pretty helpless.

This I know, though: Every new limitation is a new challenge. When my body was young and supple, I could do
with it whatever I wanted to, almost. Now, suddenly, all
these restrictions. They are, however, the restrictions that
lead to creativity.

If Beethoven had not lived within the restrictions that musical form imposes, the creativity that produced those wonderful symphonies would never have been possible. If you don't believe me, just listen to some of the undisciplined "music" that surrounds us today. It is not creative because it is not first disciplined. Ted Williams and Joe Morgan and the other great baseball hitters were successful because they disciplined themselves to know when a pitch was in the strike zone, when it was a fastball and when a curve. They didn't swing at the pitches they knew they couldn't hit, so they hit more than most. They lived within their limitations, and they were successful.

Okay, the restrictions of cancer are not always pleasant or desirable. But they can lead to creativity. You have to learn new ways of doing, of being, or getting things done. If you can't get the old things done, you have to learn new things to do. If I could be out playing third base or running marathons or talking with my friends, I wouldn't be writing these words.

One of the gifts of cancer is the challenge, the challenge to live within new limitations, to have our lives renewed at the very moment we are dis-eased. That, after all, is what a challenge is, being at dis-ease with what has been, so that something new can take its place.

Harry Houdini, the great escape artist, used to say, "The smaller the box, the greater the escape."

I'm learning what it is to have a part of my body burned out to make room for the spirit to grow.

Now that I have cancer,
I'm learning to live with limits.

... I make sure I know where I am.

N O ONE ELSE DOES.
That's overstating the case a bit. My wife and children know where I am. Many of my friends do. The dog always does when she wants a snack. I'm sure God does.

But my doctor didn't! The day after my operation, my surgeon went on vacation. That's fine; I like for surgeons to be well rested. His partner came to see me while he was out of town. When he returned to the hospital, however, the partner stopped coming. My doctor didn't show up, either.

I was supposed to be moving from clear liquids to full liquids to a solid diet, but they had me stuck on the clear stuff. You know, the grape juice they strain through nuclear waste to give it that special taste. I was getting light-headed and nauseous from lack of food, but the nurses said they couldn't move me up on the food chain because the doctors had written no new orders. Finally, when I got that story one night about 8:30, I wailed, "But the doctors couldn't write any new orders. They haven't been in for three days."

"Three days? Are you sure?"

It was actually only about two and a half, but for the first time since I was wheeled into the hospital, I sensed I had the serve. I wasn't going to lose it over twelve hours of night.

"Yes, three," I said. "Maybe they died. Maybe their AA meeting ran long. Maybe they moved and didn't tell anyone. Aren't they required to give two weeks notice if they quit?"

I was enjoying this. I was on a roll. So was Paula, the night nurse. It was a delight to see her hustle out of the room to phone those doctors. All of a sudden I realized it: I had control!

She returned and said, "The kitchen is closed, but they said you can have whatever we've got, which is ice cream and graham crackers."

"You mean I can go straight from that awful grape juice to ice cream?"

"They said you can try anything. If you keep it down, you can go home. I think they feel a little guilty. Your surgeon forgot you were here."

That ice cream just about gagged me, but I shambled through the halls all night, willing it to stay where it was. It did. I went home.

He forgot I was there! My own surgeon, who rightly has a reputation as one of the best around, who knows my insides more intimately than anyone but God, forgot I was in the hospital! He didn't know I was there.

I thought all I had to do was lie there, and someone would take care of me. It wouldn't require any thought or action from me at all. Not so, I found. It's my life. I've got to take care of it. I'm the only one who really knows where I am.

I guess I am in that middle 70 percent that has to be taught to take control of our own lives. There is a 15 percent group that does it automatically. They're the aggressive type; it's a good type to be when you are sick. There is another 15 percent that just rolls over and dies, regardless of what anyone tries to do for them. We middle 70 percent can take control, can be responsible for ourselves, but we have to learn to do it.

Now I thank God that my surgeon forgot where I was. His forgetfulness gave me a great gift, the gift of control, the responsibility for my own wellness.

We can't just sit back and expect someone else to do it. Sure, we all need help. I couldn't have operated on myself. I couldn't prescribe chemo for myself. There are days I can't do anything by myself. But I am the one who has to know where I am, and where I want to be. Otherwise, I won't be there.

Now that I have cancer,
I make sure I know where I am.

. . . I'm in a prison of pain.

I CAN'T COMMUNICATE ABOUT IT, and I can't admit anyone else into it. Others cannot get into my cell even if they wish to. The pain is a wall between us. We might as well be in separate worlds.

The rule of ninety and ten applies. In major surgery, the patient's life is changed 90 percent. The patient retains only 10 percent contact with his former life. Those around him are changed only 10 percent by the surgery; they retain 90 percent of their former lives—jobs, household chores, regular routines.

I can interact only with and to pain, and to 10 percent of the life of those around me. Thus they end up ignoring me and relating to one another because it is more natural for them; they still share 90 percent with one another, only 10 percent with me. They talk about me. They talk to one another. Rarely do they talk to me.

So I have become a management problem, rather than a person—to the hospital, to my family, to visitors. They see me in my pain and don't know what to do about it. They've never seen me this way before. I understand, but it hurts—not just the pain, but not being a person.

When we are sick, we are overwhelmed by the illness. It becomes our only reality. It's not that we have a clear focus and thus don't see the rest of the world around us, like an athlete who shuts out the crowd noise as she concentrates on the point where the racket smacks the ball. It's more like being in a thick fog, so that we have no focus at all. When you are in pain, the pain takes over. You can't think about anything else. You can't think at all; you can only feel.

I believe that's why we get so spiritual at times like this, so "religious," if you will. I know I've "gotten religion," which is an especially ironic thing for me to say, since I've spent my adult life being religious as a profession. But it's like Peter O'Toole's protest in the film *My Favorite Year*, when his character learned he would have to go on live: "But I'm not an actor; I'm a movie star!" When it comes to facing pain, none of us is anything but amateur.

Thinking is about beliefs, doctrines, ideas—things of the head. Feeling is about pain and joy—things of the heart. Feeling is spiritual, it digs deep into the heart of truth that cannot be spoken but only experienced. When you are in pain—the pain of surgery and cancer and being a problem instead of a person—thinking drops off and feeling takes over.

Feeling also makes us individuals, just as pain does. No one can share the pain. Neither can anyone tell us how to feel, what is right or wrong to feel. We simply feel whatever we feel, that's all there is to it, be it despair or elation, pain or joy, fear or faith.

It is strange how pain makes us more individual. We are actually more reliant on others physically. We need their care for our bodies, their pain pills and wet cloths. But we have to become more reliant on ourselves spiritually. At the very time others are treating us more as nonpersons because we no longer share their world, at least during the time of our pain, we actually become more real as persons because we are more individual, spiritual, unique.

We are so used to thinking, however, instead of feeling, that it is hard for us to accept this. Our brains use up all their energy on pain, so we assume nothing significant can come of it. Most of the time we don't even know how we feel. That's why pain takes us over so completely—it requires us to feel instead of to think. It requires us to be spiritual persons instead of social persons.

> *Now that I have cancer, I'm in a prison of pain.*
> *That is also a cell of uniqueness, of feeling, of*
> *spirituality. I'm released from thought to walk*
> *in the fog and feel its soft and shifting contact.*
> *I am a unique person because the pain I feel*
> *is mine alone.*

WHEN
IT'S TIME
TO FIGHT

... It's "no more Mr. Nice Guy."

I DON'T WANT TO BE WELL ADJUSTED to the diagnosis, to my cancer. I don't want to be a "good patient." I don't want my doctor and the chemo nurses and whoever else I deal with to think I'm "nice" and "cooperative." I don't want to be a pain, but I don't want to have a pain, either. The well-adjusted don't survive.

The problem is, I don't know how to be anything but nice. I've always been nice. I learned early that you get rewarded for being nice, or at least that you stay out of trouble that way.

I heard a story of a court case. An Amish farmer was suing for damages. It seems a car had collided with his buggy. The judge asked him why he was suing since he had told the investigating police officer at the time of the accident that he wasn't hurt.

"Well," said the farmer, "he went over to my horse. He said, 'This horse is hurt,' and he shot it. Then he went over to my dog. He said, 'This dog is hurt,' and he shot it. Then he came over to me and said, 'Are you hurt?' and I said, 'No, sir!'"

It makes good sense, doesn't it? If you think someone is going to shoot you if you show any hurt, any vulnerability, then you keep saying, "No, sir! Nothing wrong with me. . . ." But there are things wrong. There are real hurts in our lives, and they don't get better because we keep them out of sight.

There's a line in the song "Sixteen Tons" that says "Trouble and fightin' are my middle name." I admire that ornery coal miner. I wish "trouble and fightin'" were my middle name. Instead, my middle name is "suppression and fear." (I'll never get a country-western song written about me if I can't get a more lyrical middle name than that!)

What's your middle name? I'll bet it's something like mine, because cancer patients are notorious emotion suppressers. We're like the man who caught the porcupine under a tub. You've got a darn mad porcupine under there, and no idea which way it'll come out if you don't hold it down. So you just keep sitting on the tub.

Most of us cancer patients get so many porcupines down inside, the really prickly kind, usually without even knowing it. The porcupines don't have any place to go, so they get together and build a tumor just to have a place to hang out.

The tumor gets cut out, or radiated, or flushed out with chemicals, but that doesn't solve the porcupine problem. That just gets rid of the hangout. They'll build another one if we still try to keep them under the tub, if we don't let them leave.

I'm doing better with the porcupine problem. I cry more now. I laugh more, too. If people ask me how I feel, and I feel rotten that day, I don't smile and say, "Oh, just fine." I tell them I feel rotten. (One of the reasons I laugh more now is the expressions on their faces when I tell it like it is.) I see a psychologist; I read that cancer patients who do that have twice as good a survival rate. I'm learning to be honest with her about how I really feel. In fact, I'm learning to be honest with myself.

Every once in a while, I pull up a porcupine that blinks and says, "Whee! Why didn't you let me out of there before?" We both feel better when it's gone.

So, look out, world. No more Mr. Nice Guy here. Now that I have cancer, my middle name is "getting sort of honest." It's still not good enough for a song, but keep listening to your radio. . . .

Now that I have cancer,
it's "no more Mr. Nice Guy."

. . . I believe in old clichés . . .

THAT FORMERLY I SCORNED. "When the going gets tough, the tough get going." "Today is the first day of the rest of your life." "I have cancer, but cancer doesn't have me." "No day is over if it makes a memory." "Not everyone will be cured, but everyone can be healed." "There's no problem so great that God and I together can't solve it."

To the uninitiated, they sound like so many bumper stickers. You can't help but be a little cynical about people who live by such simplistic slogans, can you?

My cancer friend, Jean Cramer-Heuerman, whose wisdom and insight appear often in these meditations, used to sit beside me at meetings. Together we laughed behind our hands when someone pulled out one of the old chestnuts. We preferred long and complicated arguments that acknowledged the intricacies that really do inhabit every human situation. (See, you can tell by that sentence!) If we had a slogan, it was Oliver Wendell Holmes's statement: "I'd give anything for the simplicity on the far side of complexity, but nothing for the simplicity on the near side of complexity." Now, even that one takes on new meaning!

Then Jean and I got cancer about the same time. She says that when you get cancer, suddenly there is new life in the old clichés. It's a form of emotional recycling.

What does it take to deal with cancer? The experts tell us the answer is in four words—three Cs and an S.

The first C is Challenge. You have to accept the challenge cancer gives. In other words, "When the going gets tough, the tough get going." "There's no problem so great that God and I together can't solve it." "Your disability is your opportunity."

The second C is Control. You can't just think of yourself as a victim. In other words, "I have cancer, but cancer doesn't have me." "No day is over if it makes a memory." "Cancer is not a sentence, just a word."

The third C is Commitment, involvement: "Today is the first day of the rest of your life." "Not everyone will be cured, but everyone can be healed." "I believe." "Be patient with me; God isn't finished yet."

The S is Support: "Jesus loves me, this I know, for the Bible tells me so." "I get by with a little help from my friends." "God made me, and God doesn't make junk."

Well, there you have it. Simple, isn't it? Just take cancer, stir in some old clichés, and you have a recipe for getting by, "one day at a time."

What's your favorite? Just write it in here. . . .

Now that I have cancer, I believe in the old clichés. When you have cancer, they are not clichés anymore, though, are they?

... *Baseball is my favorite game.*

MAYBE IT ALWAYS WAS. For an old guy, I still have great reflexes. I even stand in front of the mirror every day to admire my reflexes. I play the closest third base of any "hot corner" fielder in the Rocking Chair League. I've got the reflexes and the guts. (I've also got such a weak arm that I have to be halfway to first base when I field a ball or I can't "peg" it over there.) Being a little stupid doesn't hurt any, either, if you're going to play that close.

I love basketball, too, almost as much as I love chocolate-covered graham crackers. Football is fun, if you like to see big people playing "king of the hill" without a hill. I get a kick out of soccer. But baseball is definitely my favorite now, because time never runs out as long as you have left even one swing at the ball.

The trouble with basketball and football and soccer and most other games is that they have time limits. When the sixty minutes or the forty minutes have ticked off, that mournful whistle blows. The game is over.

Take football. Football coaches are like oncologists who think they are realists. They pace the sidelines and say, "Only five more minutes." When the game goes into overtime, the loser is subject to "sudden death." Who wants to watch football and cancer at the same time?

But baseball! As that great baseball philosopher, Yogi Berra, once said, "It ain't over till it's over." Most people think Yogi's dike has a leak when he makes statements like that. You see, though, Yogi is thinking with that baseball mentality. It ain't over when the time runs out. It's only over when the last out is made. You can be down nineteen to one, but as long as you have one more swing, you know you can win. Bottom of the ninth, two out, two strikes on you, down nineteen runs, and you know it ain't over yet!

I come from a long line of baseball players and Cincinnati Reds fans. My great-uncle, Rufus McFarland, played as a boy in Oakland City, Indiana, with Edd Roush, the Reds Hall of Famer. Edd's twin brother, Fred, was one of my coaches when I was a kid, and Edd sometimes came out to the field to hit line drives to us. Uncle Rufus and Edd went up the minors together. A left-side infielder at five feet, three inches, Uncle Rufus figured he would be the shortest man ever to play in the major leagues. Unfortunately, no one wanted a shortstop who really was.

That's a great heritage for a cancer patient. When I'm feeling down, I just play a little baseball. Uncle Rufus and Edd Roush and Pete Rose and Joe Morgan and Johnny Bench—all on my side, you bet! We come to bat in the bottom of the ninth and start swinging. You should see the looks of despair on the faces of the cancer team! They know, as surely as we do, that "it ain't over till it's over." In fact, we know "it ain't over even when it's over."

Thank you, Yogi. We're up. . . .

> *Now that I have cancer,*
> *baseball is my favorite game.*

. . . I'm accepting the challenge.

I F YOU'VE READ THE MEDITATION on "living within limits," you've already heard me say that I think the challenge cancer brings is one of its "gifts." Any gift, however, is just an offer, until it is accepted. Then it becomes a gift. To be healed, we have to accept the gift of challenge.

Some people have no trouble with that at all. They're always ready for a fight. They have to win regardless of the cost. That's not a bad attitude when cancer comes. Cancer throws down the gauntlet and the competitors snatch it up before it hits the ground.

Some folks give in and give up as quickly as the competitors jump into the fray. They hear the word "cancer" and just roll over. "What's the use?" they say. "Nothing I can do will make a difference." (If you think you're in this group, take a look at the meditation entitled "Cancer is the answer" on page 4. If you've already read it, it's okay to read it again.)

Most of us, though, are confused. We don't know what to do or how to do it. Fortunately, when the fog of confusion clears a little, we can be taught. We just have to learn that it's all right to accept the challenge.

I've had to learn. I like to compete, in games, but cancer's not a game. I'm not an automatic fighter, but I'm learning to take the challenge. Cancer says, "I'm betting you won't fight." I'm saying back, "In your face! You've got a battle now. . . ."

That's what cancer is—a challenge, a slap in the face

with a white glove, a summons to a duel. Cancer has done the slapping. Now, according to the ancient rules of duels, we get to choose the weapons.

So I choose—chemotherapy at close quarters . . . laser swords (radiation) at three feet . . . my hope against cancer's fear . . . my family and friends and nurses and physicians against cancer's sneaky doubts . . . the God of the Eternal Present against cancer's claim that death ends time . . . love against cancer's destruction . . . .

One of the marks of a long-term survivor is a sense of purpose in life, a new meaning for life—not in spite of the disease, but because of it. Facing down cancer is itself a reason to live.

In one way, of course, a challenge is just an opportunity to fail. What if I accept the challenge but lose the battle? Well, I figure there's no way that can happen, because the victory comes simply in taking the challenge, in not backing down. Here's a little poem:

> Love and I
> looked death in the eye.
> Death blinked.

That's what always happens. Cancer and death are hollow blusterers. They have power only to cause pain and rot to the body. They can't even touch love. The challenge is to choose love, to choose spirit, instead of giving in to fear. When we seize the challenge and shake it by the throat, we have already won.

Tom Dooley, the young medical doctor who worked in Laos in the 1950s, had a dream while in the hospital for cancer treatments. "The mountain in my dream was burned, and now they were planting the new life into the near-dead soil. . . . There was no more self-sadness, no darkness deep inside: no gritty annoyance at anyone or anything. No anger at God for my cancer, no hostility to anyone. I was out of the fog of confusion—standing under the clear light of duty."

Here was a man who knew he was going to die, that his days were numbered on the hands. Still, he accepted the challenge of what that meant. Such a person can never be a failure.

Frankly, if I were cancer, I'd be quaking in my boots. Old Cancer picked the wrong target this time! I'm going to beat this blunderer whether I live or whether I die, because Love is on my side. The only allies cancer has are doubt and fear. They don't have a chance.

Now that I have cancer, I'm accepting the challenge.

. . . I get cards.

PEOPLE SEND ME ALL SORTS OF CARDS. Funny cards. Sentimental cards. Religious cards. I like to get the cards, even when I'm so weak my wife has to read them to me. Even when my hands are so swollen and sore from chemo that I can't open them myself.

Helen taped them to the wall in my hospital room, down at the foot of the bed, where I could see them. One was huge, twelve inches by twenty-four inches. It showed a frightening nurse with a huge needle coming right toward me. I left it there because she made the real nurses and the real needles look so much better! More importantly, that wall reminded me that I had a world outside of the hospital, a world of people who prayed for me and really cared what happened to me.

My first hospital roommate kept a chain saw in bed with him. All night long he tried to start it, without success. My wife claimed he was snoring, but I still hold to the chain saw theory. When he jerked an especially explosive pull on the rope and would almost get it going, I would wake up. In the dim light from the hallway I could see my cards on the wall. Even at three in the morning, those cards reminded me that someone, somewhere, in another time zone or aroused by another chain saw (or maybe the same one), was awake and praying for me.

I think the card itself is a prayer, whether the sender means it that way or not. A card says to the sick person, I care. A prayer, after all, is just a way of saying to the universe: I care.

We can say that in various ways to the sick person, sometimes with words, sometimes with actions. People do things for me—bring me flowers or books, come and spend some time with me, relieve my wife so she can go out for a while, fill in for me on the job, take me to a chemo treatment. Somehow, though, that doesn't seem enough for one we love. There aren't enough of those little tasks to go around, anyway. We grope about for some greater way to reach out with some of our own strength, our own wholeness, our own health—to the one who's sick. We shout toward the sky: I care about what happens to this person!

Someone has said that when we stand before the judgment seat, the question we'll be asked is not "Did you believe?" but "Did you care?" That's why even "nonbelievers" pray for those they love.

Prayer isn't telling God or anyone else what to do or how to do it. None of us is smart enough for that.

Monica of ancient Hippo was a religious woman. Her son, Augustine, wanted to go to Rome, because he was a playboy and interested only in his own pleasure. Rome was the place "where it was happenin'." Monica prayed and prayed that her son would not be allowed to make his way to the fleshpots of Rome, for she was sure he would be ruined there. Augustine went anyway. There he heard Ambrose preach, and he was converted. The playboy became the saint.

Was Monica's prayer "answered"? No, not if you mean getting that for which she prayed. But her real prayer was answered. She had cried out, "I care about this boy," and God answered, "So do I."

With either a card or a prayer, it is difficult to know just what to say. What are the right words *to* one who is sick?

We're not sure, so we get a card to say it for us. What are the right words *for* one who is sick, to say to God, to shout to the universe? We're not sure about that, either, so we intone or mumble or cry out our prayers—some comical, some religious, some sentimental, just like cards.

The cards and the prayers both say: I care.

I have so many cards that if I set them on fire, they'd keep me warm the rest of my life. That's true with prayers, too. I'm blessed and supported by those who pray for me. I can feel those "spirit cards" in my soul.

They say that to get well you need three *C* words and one *S* word—Commitment, Challenge, Control, and Support. Maybe the *S* is a *C*, also—Caring.

Now that I have cancer, I get cards. . . .

. . . I'm in control.

I'M IN CONTROL OF MY LIFE, more than I've ever been before.

Sounds strange, doesn't it? You don't have much control of your life when you're a statistic, and I'm definitely a statistic. I'm in that group that has a "70 percent chance of being dead in one to two years." When they put a percentage on you, you're a statistic.

My wife's favorite way of explaining me is to shake her head in what I hope is *mock* disgust and say, "He's totally out of control." It's the funniest thing, but whenever she says that is when I'm most totally *in* control. I'm in *my* control, singing, laughing, dancing—what *I* want to do, affirming my life.

There are two ways that we get out of control. One is when we lose self-control, when we are driven by forces we don't understand and which we can't harness, when we are dragged helplessly behind the wild and raging horses of the emotions. The other is when we break free from the suffocating control that the dead hand of tradition and social expectation wraps around our throat.

In our society, ironically, when we say someone is out of control, we usually mean that person is under self-control, free both from the whirlwind forces on the inside and the brick fences that surround us on the outside.

One of the worst things a sports commentator can say about a ballplayer is that she or he "plays out of control." That means either the player is trying to go beyond the limits of her ability, or that he's straying from the coach's game plan.

When it's down to the final minute, however, and the game is on the line, the *best* thing the same commentator can say is that "he stepped up and took control." There is a time when you have to go beyond your own limits, when you have to "play above your head," when you dump the game plan and start creating something so unexpected that it will turn defeat into victory. You have to play out of control.

Cancer's like that, I think. The game is there, to be won or lost, now. Those around us still want to control us, even in cancer time. They praise us if we don't complain or admit that we hurt. They want us to be "good" patients, which means good victims. They don't want to be bothered or embarrassed by our struggles, by our wild attempts to play out of control. They don't think of it this way, but they'd rather see us lose the game than embarrass ourselves, and them, by trying in some unruly fashion to win.

There's a phrase from sports that's important to us here, though. It's called "winning ugly." You look more like Mickey Mouse than Michael Jordan, but you get the ball through the hoop anyway. You swing more like "The Born Loser" than like Ted Williams, but you still get the hit. You don't win pretty, but you win.

I have wondered about a seeming contradiction in the cancer literature I have read. One study shows that patients who participate in volunteer service to others recover better than those who don't. Another study indicates that those most free about saying "no" when asked to do something for others recover better.

I think the contradiction is solved by this matter of control. If one is really a volunteer, working to help others because that is a free choice, then that person has control. If, on the other hand, you are coerced or shamed into doing for others, be they family or friends or strangers, the control is taken away from you. We recover better if we have control, regardless of what that means about doing things for others.

To win the cancer battle, along with Commitment, Challenge, and Support, we need Control. That means we need both to be in control and to be out of control.

We need to be out of control—out of the control of others, out of the control of our own fears and greed for life. When we're out of control, that's when we're in control.

Now that I have cancer, I'm in control.

. . . *I'm committed.*

THERE ARE PROBABLY THOSE WHO THINK I ought to be "committed," like to an institution, but that's not what I mean.

Support, Control, Challenge—and Commitment, the four necessities for recovery. Commitment to self-growth and self-wellness, and commitment to something beyond, some greater growth and greater wellness, as well.

Commitment means action, a plan, doing something to get results. You can be in favor of something, but not committed to it. Democracy, for instance. I can say I'm all for democracy, but if I don't vote, I'm not committed to it. I might think it's a good idea to help the hungry, but until I give money or volunteer at a food pantry or lobby my congressman, I'm not really committed to easing the pangs of hunger.

To resist cancer, I have to take action against it, and it has to be *my* action, not someone else's. I realize that surgery or chemotherapy or radiation is my action in a very real sense, because it's my decision. In the actual doing, however, it is the action of others—researchers and pharmacists and nurses and physicians. If I stop at only cooperating with or accepting their actions, I haven't really made the commitment to fighting cancer.

Every day, Emmett Kelly, the sad-faced clown, comes and sweeps all the cancer cells out of my body. Remember his little broom? I call it the "light" broom. Actually there was a circle of light on the floor. As Kelly swept, the electrical technician made the circle smaller and smaller, mak-

44

ing it appear that the clown's broom was actually sweeping up the light. While I'm in the bathtub, I have Emmett go through my whole body, sweeping with his little circle of light. (If you've read the meditation on singing on page 13, you'll remember that visualization and music can work together nicely.) By the time he's done, all the cancer cells are gone. That visualization is something I do, that no one else can do for me.

We are really committed when we take the actions that are available to us alone—visualization, meditation, biofeedback, attending healing services, talking to ourselves, learning more about our disease and treatment so we have better control, body monitoring, prayer, giving ourselves the right messages for health, eating correctly, exercising, avoiding tobacco and alcohol, finding occasions for laughter each day, reducing stress, laying healing hands on our own bodies. . . .

Not all of these are for everyone. The more of them that we can do for ourselves, however, the greater our own sense of commitment, and the better we then feel about ourselves. That in turn increases the peace and reduces the stress in our bodies, allowing our healing agents room to work.

Research was done on women having breast biopsies. The group that reacted best was those whose first action and attitude were prayer. Faith, whether religious or otherwise, provides control. The faith of these women gave them control, which allowed them to make the commitment to action in prayer. That action reduced the level of stress hormones.

Another way the stress hormones are reduced is involvement with helping others—in a support group, in volunteer work, in someone's personal care. The way to health is not only commitment to doing the things that get me well, but commitment to action that makes healthy the society and environment around me.

Commitment is determination and action stuck together, like peanut butter and bread. It is both seeing the goal and kicking the ball toward it.

I used to run with a young woman who liked everything about running . . . except running. She was great at talking about it, reading running magazines, buying running clothes and shoes, stretching out. When it came to hitting the road, though, she didn't really want to do it. She liked the idea, but she wasn't committed.

Getting well takes commitment, which isn't easy. It surely is rewarding, though!

Now that I have cancer, I'm committed.

... I am whole.

A T LEAST, MORE WHOLE THAN I'VE BEEN BEFORE. On the face (or the colon) of it, that sounds silly. "Hole" looks more accurate than "whole." After all, a part of me is missing. Strangely now, however, I am more whole.

Connectedness is the key to wellness. Connectedness to others, to one's own self, to purpose. In other words, wholeness—putting it all together.

The less connected we are, the less together, the less whole and well we are. All those parts of us that are not integrated into the whole have more chance of getting sick, because they're out there by themselves, with no support, no surrounding buttresses of love and solidarity.

There's a story about a man who fell into the river. An old sailor rowed out to him. Just as the man was about to go under, the sailor grabbed his arm. But it was an artificial arm, and came off in the sailor's hands. The man went under again, but when he came up, the sailor grabbed his hair. Unfortunately, the man wore a wig, and it, too, came off in his hands. When the man rose yet once again, the old salt grabbed his clothes and shouted, "How can I save you if you won't stick together?"

We've got to stick together if we want to get well. That means we integrate mind, body, and spirit. The best mark of a long-term survivor is the integration—into wholeness—of love and attitude and looking for purpose and exercise and diet and spirituality and laughter and appreciation for life and relationships and self-love and seeing new options and learning new ways.

We don't have to have all these in place when we start. They are all approaches that can be learned. Wellness is often a matter of finding new options, seeing in ways we haven't been trained to see. Working hard at learning and integration does the immune system more good than any other therapy.

Cancer is a spiritual disease because it requires us to face the dilemma of fragmentation and wholeness. In our culture we are used to the adversarial system, whether it is lawyer vs. lawyer in the justice system, cop vs. criminal on the streets, cowboy vs. Indian in the movies, man vs. woman in marriage, team vs. team on the athletic field, management vs. labor in the workplace. There must be a loser for each winner. Someone has to be "number one," and that's the only number that counts.

In trying to beat cancer, however, I am competing against myself. Cancer is a part of me, so if I win, I also lose. Getting whole, getting well, has to do with oneness. It's not a matter of right or wrong, victory or defeat, not even life or death. It is life vs. nonlife. If I experience wholeness in life, death is not a defeat. If I experience fragmentation in life, then life is not a victory.

The goal, the sense of purpose, is not so much getting cured, beating the cancer, continuing to live. The goal is wholeness itself, being a full and complete person. That is adequate purpose. In fact, it is the only worthy purpose of life. I don't have to make some great achievement, do some mighty work, to justify my existence. Being a whole person *is* the purpose for our being.

There is no single road to wellness. Getting well and being well is taking an interlocking network of highways that lead to the one, central junction of wholeness.

Cure is an end-result concept. Wellness, health, healing, wholeness—these are process, each-moment-at-a-time concepts. I don't just want to be cured, to reach the end of one road. I want to be whole for each moment of all my life, whether my days are few or many.

Sickness, especially from cancer, often produces spirituality. One reason is because we are taught visualization and meditation and prayer as methods for increasing our body's healing agents, enhancing our immune system. I think there's something spiritual about cancer itself, though. It's a challenge to wholeness, to the integration of love. If we take the challenge of cancer, we almost have to face our fragmentation and begin to pull together the scattered pieces of our selves.

Now that I have cancer, I am whole.

. . . I've got an attitude.

THEY SAY YOU HAVE A BETTER CHANCE if you have a good attitude. I'm not sure about that. I suspect the most important thing is just to have an attitude. Your own attitude. Period.

There is a man in my support group. His name is Jim. He's had cancer twice. They told him the first time he wouldn't live a year. The second time he lost a lung. He's convinced he'll get it a third time—if he lives that long. He's been going around with a bad attitude for five years. He's proud of it.

"They say you've got to have a good attitude. Ridiculous! I've got the worst attitude there is, and I'm still here!"

Jim really grooves on "havin' a 'tude," as the saying goes. He doesn't feel the need for any "attitude adjustment," either. He's baaaaad . . . and he's glaaaaad!

Jim doesn't have what anyone could describe as a "good" attitude, but he has a great attitude for dealing with cancer. He's so proud of living with a bad one that he keeps on going just to prove it can be done. It gives him a reason to keep fighting. He's got a cause. He's accepted the challenge. He's made the commitment. He's out to prove you don't have to have a good attitude to deal with cancer, which is a good attitude to take. He'll do it even if it means he has to live.

What we really need is a cancer attitude, not a good attitude. "Anything that works," that's the cancer motto. Cancer is a very personal disease. Each of us must deal with it in his or her own best way.

Bernie Siegel says he can always tell when a patient is

going to get well. It's when a nurse or another physician has marked "Bad Attitude" on the chart. It means the patient is taking responsibility. In other words, the patient is not being "cooperative," isn't doing what makes life easier for the nurses and technicians and physicians.

I'm very open about having cancer, and about my treatment, and about my pains, and about . . . well, just everything about the disease. That's difficult for some people. It scares them. They don't even want to hear the word, yet alone hear about what it's like.

One man told me about his friend, "Dan."

"Dan," he said, "got cancer, but he never talked about it. Why, you'd never even know he had it. He just went right on with life as usual."

"He sounds like a good man," I said. "I'd like to meet him."

"Uh, well, you can't. He's dead . . . but you'd never know he had it, right up to the day he died."

With no blame on Dan, he's not a good model for me. I don't want to be like him. He's dead.

How many times have you heard an ill person, whether with cancer or arthritis or another debilitating disease, extolled in words like these: "Oh, she never complains. Even when she's feeling her worst, if you ask her how she is, she always smiles and replies, 'Just fine.'"

I'm not going to argue with those folks. Like I said, it's a personal disease. Each of us has to take the attitude we think is best for us. If you say "I'm just fine," when you're hurting, that's just fine, as long as it's your decision, your real attitude. But is it your decision? Is it your attitude, or is it the attitude someone else has decided you ought to take?

I admire folks who do the best they can with what

they've got, even if it's not much. There's a way in which each of us ought to be able to say "Just fine," regardless of how much we're hurting. "Just fine" is a relative term. My condition might not be acceptable for you, but it's "just fine" for me.

That is for me to decide, though, for me—and for you to decide for you. The best attitude is the one that is true and genuine, the one that really is mine, the one that really is yours—not the one that is the most convenient and non-threatening for others.

Now that I have cancer,
I've got an attitude . . . and it's mine.

WHEN
YOU'RE BALD
AND STRANGELY
BEAUTIFUL

. . . I'm my own hero.

BERNIE SIEGEL says that disease gives us a chance to live out our personal myths and become heroes. I have many personal myths—baseball star, jazz bassoonist, great writer. The most enduring one, though, is that I am a runner.

I've always thought of myself as a long-distance runner. I've not always been one, you understand, but I've always thought of myself that way! In grade school, I thrilled as Glenn Cunningham made his assaults on the "unbreakable" four minute barrier for the mile run. In those days, a mile was considered long-distance running by most people. When I went out for track in high school, I decided to double the heroics by running the two-mile race. Later, as a road runner, ten kilometer (6.2 miles) races were popular. Gradually I worked up to the marathon—26 miles, 385 yards.

We distance runners are, on the whole, a disdainful lot. We like to say things like: "Oh, you need me there in thirty minutes and it's ten miles? Well, my wife has the car, but I'll just run over." (Don't bother to figure up the arithmetic; it will only confuse you!) Or we put slogans on our shirts like, "When the going gets tough, the sprinters stop." We tend to think that our many miles will save us from all health problems, except sore feet, shin splints, aching joints, and sagging breasts, of course. We assume we'll never die; we'll just run off into the sunset some day and not return. We are, quite simply, arrogant in our health. We work at it, but we assume that work is a guarantee. Consequently, we're not prepared when our bodies get cancer or heart disease. "But look at all those miles I put in," we want to wail.

Now I find those miles work for me in a different way. With a chemo habit on my back and a Groshong catheter in my chest, I'm just a slow walker these days, not the distance runner I thought I was. But I *have* been there. I have seen the finish line after twenty-six miles. I know I can do a marathon, because I have done a marathon.

So I divided my fifty-two weeks of chemotherapy up into fifty-two one-half-mile segments of a marathon. I said to myself, "I know I can complete this chemo course, because I can complete any marathon course." Half mile by half mile, I have done it. I know what it is to "hit the wall," in either marathon. I know what it is to ache so bad that all I want to do is quit, in either marathon. But I have run them both, and I have finished the course.

> *I've always thought of myself as a long-distance*
> *runner. Now that I have cancer, I think of myself*
> *as a long-distance victor. And a hero.*

. . . *I'm superstitious.*

I'VE NEVER BEEN SUPERSTITIOUS BEFORE. Oh, I always wear my Hoosiers cap with the bill cocked to the left when I watch Indiana University basketball games, but that's just fun. I don't really think it affects the score. Now, however, I want so much to do the "right" things and avoid the "wrong" things—the actions and even the thoughts that might determine whether my cancer goes or stays.

When I go in for a chemo treatment, I sit in the chair where my vein puckered up best to take the IV needle. I know the chair didn't have anything to do with it, but I'm taking no chances. I had a banana for breakfast before my last chemo treatment, and I didn't get sick. I've had so many breakfast bananas since that I'm beginning to walk like a chimp. Maybe bananas are just good sense instead of superstition. But what about the plaid shirt phenomenon? I don't get mouth sores on days I wear plaid to chemo. You think I'm going to take a chance on a plain shirt? No way!

I'm an amateur magician. I love to make children laugh and wonder how in the world I made the three ropes one, or made the ball disappear and then come out Patty's ear. Magic is fun. It's not wise to take it seriously, though. I can't put cancer into my red velvet bag and make it go away. I can't cause it to disappear up my sleeve by saying "Abracadabra."

So what's the difference between being superstitious and simply acknowledging the mysterious nature of life? Where does faith trail off into magic? What is good sense and what is just silliness? What is "the right thing"?

I'm not sure there is a right thing—a right chair to sit in, or shirt to wear, or even right food to eat. But if there is no right thing to do, how will I get well? Is my health really just a matter of chance? Is there nothing I can do to help?

I suspect there are "right" things to do, but they are not in the realm of chairs or shirts, or even bananas. They have more to do with faith than magic, prayer than potions, good thoughts than correct rituals. Sometimes, though, we need to express our own faith in the future, and in the present, by acting out our fears and hopes. If I wear a plaid shirt and sit in the same chair each time in the chemo room, I'm saying that I'm not just a victim. I'm not a withering leaf, blown by whatever wind has the most bluster. I have choices to make, and those choices make a difference.

I can choose love instead of fear, wholeness rather than fragmentation, relationship over loneliness, control instead of dependence. Those choices are never easy, but they are possible. One way I remind myself that I can make those choices is by which shirt I wear and which chair I sit in. My superstitions are signs of hope.

Now that I have cancer,
I'm superstitious . . . and hopeful.

. . . I'm waiting for "the last drop on the last day."

THAT'S THE ONE, my oncologist assures me, that makes the cure.

Of course, my oncologist is a bit of a comedian. "Does it hurt yet?" he asks me as he installs the Groshong catheter in my chest. "No," I tell him. "Darn," he says. "I must be doing something wrong." At least, I *think* he's a comedian. . . .

He keeps giving me the "last drop" theory to keep me going. My side effects were so bad the first month of chemotherapy—mouth sores to the point I couldn't eat or talk; diarrhea out the . . . well, that goes without saying; eyes watering and gluing themselves shut and going out of focus; veins inflamed; hands and feet swelling, so bad I couldn't walk for a couple of days.

One dark night at two A.M. I promised myself I could quit at the end of six months, instead of going the whole twelve, if they didn't get better. The problem is that I'm part of a clinical trial. It would mess up the statistics if I quit early. He keeps making me wait for the last drop on the last day.

I'm glad he does. I want to be part of the clinical trial. I want my pain to be useful in learning things that will be valuable in treating others.

Maxwell House used to advertise its coffee as "good to the last drop." I have no doubt that chemo will be bad to the last drop, but I'm going to keep going, and not just because I'll mess up somebody's statistics.

There's an old story from the river country close to

where I grew up. The waters rose in the spring, as they always did, flooding the countryside and driving people up onto the rooftops. One whole family was up there, watching things float by—a tree, a chicken coop, a pig, an old hat. . . . But the old hat stopped at the edge of their yard and turned around and went back upstream, against the flood. At the other edge, it stopped again, turned and came back down. Back and forth it went, with the water, then against the water, as the family sat and wondered what strange phenomenon could have caused this unlikely sight. Then one of the boys slapped his head and exclaimed, "I remember now. Grandpa said he was going to mow the yard today, come hell or high water."

There are some things that you do just because you have to. Our younger daughter, Katie, says that is the best thing I ever told her, which is pretty good considering what she usually thinks of my advice.

"You've told me a lot of lies," she says.

"What do you mean? How could I ever have told you a lie?"

"Well, for instance, you always said, 'You'll understand it better when you're older.' I'm older now, but I don't understand things any better. But when I went to college, you said, 'There are some things you have to do just because you have to do them. You don't have to feel like doing them or want to do them or have the right circumstances for doing them. You just have to do them.' That's gotten me through a lot of tough jobs."

Someone surmised to the Duke of Wellington after his defeat of Napoleon at Waterloo that the English soldiers must have been braver than the French soldiers, to have won the victory.

"No," replied Wellington, "the French soldiers were brave. But the English soldiers were brave five minutes longer."

I suspect that's often the case—not how brave or smart you are, but how long you use the intelligence and courage given you.

Now that I have cancer,
I'm going for the last drop on the last day.

. . . I'm trying to learn to be a complainer.

COMPLAINERS GET WELL BETTER. They get all their negative feelings out, get all those emotional toxins out of their system. You ever heard of a prize fighter who got cancer? Of course not. They might be a little loopy, but they don't have any aggression or hostility turned inward on themselves. They get it all out on the heads of other people.

Some complainers do that, too, which is why we're taught not to complain. So many people make complaining into a nasty business, by dumping their dis-ease all over everyone else, instead of dropping it off at the safe emotional nuclear-waste dump. So from the time we are little children, we are told we should keep a stiff upper lip, be a brave boy or girl, or a "big" one, knowing that "big" boys and girls don't cry, and not bother other people with our complaints about life.

Thank goodness Helen and I were unsuccessful with our daughters. We tried and tried to make them stoical uncomplainers. They would have nothing of it. A neighbor once named our older daughter, then about eight, "Mary Too." Mary was always too hot or too cold, too tall or too short, too hungry or too full, too rich or too poor. The world was too light or too dark. She was Mary "Too." Too much of a complainer, her parents felt, but she had built-in good instincts, for which we are very grateful. A child's good instincts make up for a lot of bad parenting.

So now I'm trying to learn from my children. I'm complaining, in safe ways and safe places. I go to cancer support group. I attend prayer circle at church. I tell God all about it. I walk it off, muttering complaints with every step. Everybody in town knows about my watery eyes. When someone asks me how I am, they find out! (If they don't want to know, they shouldn't ask.)

Even saying all that embarrasses me, though. I'm not a complaining type. I know there are so many people who have it worse than I do. What do I have to complain about? I've always gotten my points from being a "nice" person, one who caused no strain or pain to others. Down deep, I still think that's the way a person is supposed to be. But thank God for my family and friends. They say, "Hey, lean on us. You don't have to be nice all the time. We love you regardless. If you hurt, you tell us. If you don't like having cancer, good for you. Complain and get well. We'd rather have a complaining and alive you than just a 'nice' memory."

One of my chemo-pushing nurses said one day, "Now you listen. This is no competition to see who can stand the most pain. If I hurt you, you tell me." She's right, as chemo nurses always are. This isn't a "niceness" contest. This is a getting-well struggle, and I'm going to win, even if I have to kick a little . . . well, "niceness" habit.

Have I told you about my diarrhea? No? Well, just wait until you hear this. . . .

> *Now that I have cancer,*
> *I'm learning to be a complainer.*

. . . My morning misery has become a joy.

I T DIDN'T START OUT THAT WAY. In fact, I didn't even
have a morning misery until I had cancer.

I've always been a morning person. I love to get up
with the sun and the roosters, sip a cup of tea, run five
miles, have some time for myself. Unfortunately, I'm also a
night person. I love to stay up late, reading good novels and
watching bad TV. Being both a morning person and a night
person is a bad combination; it's hard to get any sleep, especially if the people who are paying you expect you to
work during the day.

Now I'm neither a morning nor a night person. I'm so
tired I can't stay up late. Sometimes I sleep ten hours and
feel no more rested when I get up than when I went to bed.
Worst of all, though, is what happens to my insides in the
morning.

They removed one-third of my colon to get that malignant tumor out, then resectioned it. That changed my
bowel habits. (Noncancer folks might think this isn't polite
to talk about, but it's the real world for us, right?) Ever
since, I get thirty to ninety seconds notice before I have to
be seated, and I don't mean at a table. When it happens, I
don't want to be very far from a bathroom!

This severely reduced bowel, what I call my semi-colon,
moves four or five times in the first three or four hours after
I get up in the morning, with no more than a warning of a
minute and a half to me. That's more movements than a
symphony! It might even be more times than that if the

chemo has given me diarrhea. In addition, in the aftermath of surgery, I've had trouble with hemorrhoids, something I never before experienced. After each movement, I have to get undressed, get in the shower, and "cleanse myself thoroughly and gently." Now with that combination, I'm sure you understand when I use the term "morning misery."

So why do I say it's a joy? Because I've gotten acquainted with Bernie Siegel and Joan Borysenko and Norman Cousins and Greg Anderson and Gerald May and Regina Sara Ryan and Mary McDermott Shideler in the process. There's a little table in my bathroom, one my father made. On it are piled their books. I don't allow myself to read them except when I'm in the bathroom. It makes me look forward to my period of morning misery.

These folks are my friends and soul physicians. They speak to me the wisdom I need to hear. Some of them I had heard of vaguely before. Others are brand new to me. Some of the books have been given to me or recommended to me by friends. Others I have found browsing bookstore shelves. (Not in the morning, of course!)

My life is so enriched by these new friends. I can't imagine what I would do without our daily chats. Each day I learn new coping skills. I learn how to live fully within the limits I'm now given. With their guidance I feel more deeply into my own life and the love that is there for me in the presence of others.

Beethoven said that if he had to choose between the joys and sorrows of his life, he would keep the sorrows, because he had learned so much more from them. I understand what he meant. If I had to lose my new friends to get rid of my morning misery, I would keep the misery!

I'm not just trying to avoid the morning misery by being

transported into the realm of books, so I can mask out what is actually happening to me. I stay in the moment, even the moment of distress. But these authors participate in the present with me. It's not avoidance of the pain and discomfort, but the misery is diminished by being shared.

I could, of course, read Bernie and Joan and Gerald and Mary and the others at some other time. That, however, would not change my morning routine, and my misery would be only that—misery.

> *I suspect it's better to have misery one can share with friends than to have joy and no one with whom to share it. That's why, now that I have cancer, my morning misery is a joy.*

. . . I get sick when I see Becky.

ECKY IS THE HEAD NURSE in the cancer clinic. She's my "pusher," inserting that needle, pushing that chemo into me. I like Becky. She's competent and pleasant and very pretty. I could look at her all day, except for one thing: She makes me sick!

You've probably heard this kind of story already, so here are some more . . .

Marie, a nurse practitioner at my cancer clinic, a lovely and sophisticated lady, came around the corner of an aisle in a grocery store one day. She came face to face with a clinic patient. The woman promptly threw up all over poor Marie!

An American oncologist walking down a street in Paris saw a woman coming toward him. She suddenly doubled up and started vomiting in the gutter. He hurried to her to see if he could help. Then he recognized her, from back in the States. She was a former chemo patient. He hadn't seen her for eight years! One look at his face, though, even in a foreign country, and there went the cookies!

I have a friend who munches crackers on her forty-five-mile drive to her chemo treatments. As soon as she gets into the car and heads north out of her town, she feels the nausea coming on. The crackers help keep it down.

So we come back to the ever-gracious Becky, who's been enduring tales like this for the fifteen years of her oncology nursing practice. I park in the garage. I walk across the street, down the stairs, into the long tunnel over to the cancer clinic. With every step the nausea level rises higher.

Finally, I walk into the clinic, see Becky, and run like mad for the restroom, to "call Ralph on the big white phone." (Isn't it amazing, the number of euphemisms we have for vomiting?)

It's called "anticipatory nausea." It reminds us that we are a unity of body and mind. Nothing has been put into my body yet, to make me sick, when I walk in and see Becky. In fact, I'm as far away from my last nauseating treatment as I'll ever be, so I ought to be at my best, right? No way! My mind knows what's coming. It has a reason, even if my body doesn't.

Some people say that it's silly to get sick, or feel pain, when your body hasn't yet been subjected to it. "It's all in your head," they say, as though what's in your head doesn't count.

What's in your head does count, and the count goes even higher when you add what's in your nose and taste buds and ears and eyes. William Redd, a psychologist who's done a great deal of research in this area, is a consultant to fragrance manufacturers. He says, "If you want to sell your perfume, don't let a nurse wear it."

There are ways we can neutralize the anticipatory nausea and pains—hypnosis, meditation, relaxation techniques, imaging. Some hospitals and cancer clinics have even begun to teach these. Probably the most simple is just to put yourself, in your mind, some place you'd rather be.

When I park in the garage now, it's the same garage I park in across from Riverfront Stadium when I go to see the Reds play. When I walk that long tunnel, it's the gangway across the street to the blue seats. Then I step into the clinic, and there they are, watching for me in the waiting room, cheering that I have finally arrived to save the game—Joe

Morgan and Chris Sabo and Johnny Bench and Pete Rose, you bet.

The mind is a great gift from God, with its ability to imagine, to be playful. If we get careless with it, it can get us into a lot of trouble, but it can also be the way of healing. Anticipatory nausea reminds us that we are whole creatures, and we need to be healed as a whole, mind and body both, together.

I'll admit that Becky looks a little strange in a Reds uniform, but at least she's not nauseating!

. . . I am blessed.

I LEARNED THAT FROM A YOUNG MAN in the cancer center. No, not a doctor, nor a nurse, nor a fellow patient. The janitor.

One nauseated and cold chemo day I left my car in the hospital parking garage and started the long walk through the underground tunnel to the cancer center. Step by step . . . I knew what was waiting. . . . Step by step, closer to the verge. . . . Yes, you know the verge I mean, "the urge to regurge," as we said as children. And not a toilet or sink in sight.

Self-pity swirled around me like a pernicious fog, the thick kind of fog the Scots call "the dreaded haar." Dread like a stone in the belly.

I was just about to decorate the wall with my breakfast when the janitor appeared from around the bend in the tunnel, pulling a big cart full of rubbish. Well, you really hate to throw up in the hallway when the one who has to clean it up is standing right there, so I took a deep breath and started to go on.

"How are you today?" he asked, eyes flashing and teeth gleaming.

It was clearly a good day for him. I resented his obvious vitality and robust health. He looked like he could eat a pickled Chevrolet and never burp. So I decided to answer his question truthfully.

We do that sometimes, don't we? We tell the truth as revenge. Like my nun friend, Sister Thecla, says: "Sing loudly. That way we can get back at God for giving us these voices."

69

People say, "How are you?" and expect to hear an automatic "Fine." Well, I wasn't "fine," and I told him so.

"I'm miserable," I mumbled.

He sobered up immediately, his ear cocked toward me like a collie. Then I felt a little guilty. After all, he was just being pleasant. It wasn't fair to put him on the spot like that.

So I did the usual. I asked him back, "How are you?"

With a remarkable combination of dignity and joy and compassion, he replied, "Blessed!"

"Blessed!" What a happy expression.

You know, it didn't do a thing for my nausea. I went on down the hall and threw up in the bathroom. I assume the blessed janitor had to clean it up.

Blessings, however, are not just a matter of how we feel at the moment, although I'll be the first to admit that a day without pain and fatigue and side effects is a blessing all by itself. The blessings are there for the taking, even if the miseries have caught us by the hair and started yanking. As I hugged the porcelain deity, I said, "Yeah, I'm blessed, even now, because God loves me, and I have people who love me. He's right. I'm blessed, too."

"Blessed." Blessed with the efforts of researchers and physicians and laboratory workers and nurses. Blessed by people who never knew me, but who taught my physicians and passed on to my nurses their caring values. Blessed with the love of people who pray for me and care for me. Whatever recovery I may have is a gift from generations of loving people. I'm blessed.

I was blessed by the truth, too. I told him how I really felt, instead of giving some glib "Okay," and it was therapeutic. Yes, sometimes we tell the truth for revenge, but saying "I'm fine" when we're not doesn't help us get well. It's the truth that makes us free to receive the blessings.

I am blessed by a young janitor, whose simple witness reminds me that life is a gift, even when I'm about to get wrung inside out by the chemo bends.

Now that I have cancer, I am blessed.

. . . I'm sick and tired of being sick and tired.

BEING TIRED DEPRESSES ME. Even the simplest tasks are hard to do. The tiredness and depression are mostly from the chemo, I know, but I have almost a year of that to go. Just about the time I get a little energy back, I have to go back for more chemo. I'm just so sick and tired of being sick and tired.

Nothing works right, either. My eyes, eyes that used to pick out a fly ball at a hundred yards, are so bad. The lids are stuck together most of the time. My friend Jack was up on the leadership platform at a meeting we both attended. I was in the front row. We've been the best of friends for years, and we weren't more than twenty feet apart, but I could barely make him out, barely pick him out from the others sitting up there.

It's not just my eyes. My hands and feet are swollen. My mouth is sore. I can't shave or use tools or go to the dentist for fear of meeting a germ or getting a cut. I spend half the day in the bathroom. If I get a whiff of the wrong smell, I'll toss my cookies. The problem is that the odors take turns being the "wrong" one. I never know which smell is the wrong one until it's too late. For two weeks after chemo I can only eat white stuff—potato soup and tapioca and crackers and pasta without sauce. I long for colored food!

I'm sick and tired of thinking about cancer, too. I'm sick of hearing about it and reading about it.

I have stacks of color-coded paper with instructions on how to deal with the side effects of my chemotherapy.

Nurses and doctors and strangers on the street give me advice and information and orders. Books and pamphlets pile up beside my place at the table, and more arrive daily in the mail.

I don't want to be a cancer expert. I just want to be done with it. I want to read Anne Tyler, not Bernie Siegel. I want to go to ball games, not support groups. Nurses are wonderful, but I never want to see a white dress again. I want to hear a mechanic say, "Your transmission's shot," rather than hear a nurse say, "This vein's shot." I want to be a good old boy and drive my pickup and drink real coffee down at the oasis and talk about the price of soybeans. I want to be "normal."

I wasn't prepared for all this. I went to get a second opinion from an oncologist who was recommended to me by a friend. For a long time they called him "Dr. Cancer," because he was the best at beating that word down. Then they got used to him so now they just call him Dr. Hatfield.

He said, "You need to be in this clinical trial, a year's worth of new chemo drugs for your type of cancer. The problem is that you have to start it within thirty days of your surgery, and this is your thirtieth day. So, take your time, and think about it, but I have to leave for a board meeting in fifteen minutes."

I just didn't get much time to get ready. I'd had no symptoms when I had the surgery. Then I had fifteen minutes to decide on chemo. I've been around cancer patients a lot in my life, but they weren't in my family, and certainly I've never been one before. I just wasn't prepared for how tired I am, how sore this is making me.

Cancer cells are fast-dividing cells. Basically the chemotherapy drugs have to attack all the fast-dividing cells, killing them all, on the theory that the healthy ones, the noncancerous ones, will regenerate. I didn't know I had so many speedy little cells—stomach and intestines and mouth and hair and palms and soles, and especially the energy cells. Those guys have really been knocked for a loop.

I think back, though, to looking for Jack, up on the platform, through my chemo-fuzzed eyes, and this is what I remember: For all the fuzziness, he still looked like my friend. It's difficult ever to have clear vision, with or without chemo. If you can recognize your friends, though, you're okay.

All those mouth sores and eye sores and foot sores—they're ways of recognizing my friends. They let me know that the chemo is doing its job, separating out the cells we don't want, letting the others have a chance to take up the room they need without being crowded out.

Now that I have cancer, I'm sick and tired of being sick and tired, but I know that, one way or another, there's a new day comin'. I'm just thankful for my friends, all of them.

. . . I'm a prisoner in my own house.

NOT ENTIRELY, of course. There are times when I must leave, most notably on those five-days-in-a-row intravenous chemotherapy weeks. There are other days when I can get out, even days when I can go to work.

But I can't be in the sunshine; the chemo's made my skin too sensitive for that. I can't go to church or to the mall or the theater if infections are lurking in the air; the chemo's suppressed my immune system too much for that. I can't hold a baby unless I've first been assured it hasn't had any recent vaccinations.

So I'm a prisoner in my own house. That bothers me. I don't want to think of my house as a prison. I like my house. It's always been a refuge, like a game preserve for an endangered species, which, perhaps, I am.

My house has big windows and lots of light. Flowering crab trees bloom just outside the glass. Squirrels and birds come right up to the ends of the branches and look in. Plants bloom around the living room. Pictures of family give me my history as I walk down the hall. Hundreds of books live here, piled on the tops of tables my father has crafted even though he's blind. Music boxes sing one to another from room to room. Puzzles and games and little horse statues remind us of when our girls still lived here. There's a grim and terrible contradiction in being a prisoner in paradise.

Sometimes now my house seems like a colonial blockhouse or western fort. I'm hunched down in here below the firing slits, trying to escape the savages that besiege our walls with their catapults and arrows and cannon. The problem is, the savages are in here, too. In fact, they are already inside of me. We're prisons within prisons. I'm a prisoner in my house, and the cancer cells are prisoners within the house of my body, trying so hard to escape that they are running rampant.

I wonder what they're so afraid of, why they started forting up in tumors, imprisoning themselves within me. Do they see the contradiction, too, of being a prisoner in a place that's meant for love and hope and beauty instead of for fear and being shut in? Prisoners and their guards always have to live together, just as the cancer cells and I do.

We are all prisoners in some way, to something. The trick of life is surely to choose your prison well. My cancer cells and I have both chosen wisely in many ways. I cannot think of a better place to be a prisoner than in my house. Apparently they could not think of a better place for imprisonment than in the house of my body.

Houses and bodies, however, are not meant to be jails. I want to be released from my house, so that it can be a home again instead of a stockade. I want my cancer cells to be freed, too. I want them to be released from the fearful compulsion that makes them multiply so quickly, so that they, also, can become normal, free, hopeful cells again and live within me as within a home rather than as bolted down and penned in, afraid of what lies outside.

> *Now that I have cancer, I'm a prisoner in my own house . . . but I have company, and we are all working to be free.*

WHEN THE NIGHT FRIGHTS COME

. . . I have to walk that lonesome valley by myself.

THAT'S WHAT THE OLD SPIRITUAL SAYS: "Jesus walked that lonesome valley, had to walk it by himself. Oh, nobody else could walk it for him . . . had to walk it by himself." Then it reminds us that each of us has to walk that lonesome valley alone as well, "have to walk it by yourself."

When I first heard that word, *cancer*, and I thought I would be dead from it very soon, the idea of walking that lonesome valley all by myself simply terrified me. I'd never thought about it before. Oh, I've certainly thought about death. You can't even see a Woody Allen movie without thinking about death. We all know that no one gets out of this life alive. But I had never realized how lonesome it would be.

I had a hospital roommate, a very nice man. Nurses and other hospital personnel streamed in and out of the room like worker ants. Friends dropped by every day, so many that my wife installed a turnstile in the doorway and made them show passes. Helen and Mary Beth and Katie must have put in twenty-four hospital hours per day between them. Still, I was in a darkening valley of pain and fear all by myself. None of those other folks, the ones in regular clothes who could eat regular food, none of them was on death's waiting list. I was the one, and it scared the hell out of me. In many ways, it still does.

That fear tells me something very important about myself. Too much of the meaning for my life comes from outside of me. I live for others—for their approval and friend-ship and affirmation. I've spent most of my life walking paths that will cause others to like me, or at least respect me. But that lonesome valley, that's one trip I've got to make all by myself. No amount of approval from others makes any difference. To negotiate that lonesome valley successfully, you've got to have your internal compass working, the one that points you straight at yourself, be-cause no one else will be there.

The results of looking away from ourselves for meaning are addictions. Addictions are always based on the mis-taken idea that we can get meaning for life from something other than our own selves, be it drugs or booze or money or sex or power or nicotine or thought patterns or exercise or rituals or food or . . . you name it. We don't sit down one day and say, "I don't think I can get meaning from my self, so I'll form an addiction to something," but that's still the reason those habits get their hold on us.

Bernie Siegel says that our pain is a reset button. If we never feel the pain, we never push the button to get our lives reset. And what is it we say about addictions? "He was feelin' no pain." The addiction masks our fear and uncer-tainty, even if it's a "positive" addiction, like reading or running or helping people or being nice. We've got to feel the pain or we don't know how we've given up all the in-ternal meaning, how we're looking to the rest of the world to make life worthwhile for us.

I think that's why Jesus was successful as a healer in some cases and not in others. Some folks were ready to have their reset buttons pushed and some were not.

Cancer has pushed my reset button. I can't live for oth-ers anymore. I don't mean I want to become selfish. There's a great difference between being self-centered and being centered in one's self. I have to be satisfied with me and my life, whether or not anyone else is.

Day by day now, I feel a little more comfortable with walking the lonesome valley by myself. I think that's a good sign. It means I'm beginning to understand that my justification for living is just that I'm here. My meaning comes from inside. All that I need for facing life, yes, and for facing death, God has already put into my life.

Now that I have cancer,
I have to walk that lonesome valley by myself.

. . . I grieve already for the loss my death will bring to the world.

THAT CERTAINLY SOUNDS like I'm entertaining a grandiose estimate of my value to the world. Not so. I'm well aware that only a precious handful will mourn my passing for very long. It is only presidents and generals, heroes and villains, composers and artists, who are remembered more than a generation, and not many of them. When my children and my tombstone have been erased by time and wind, I shall be no more to this world, not even in memory, along with billions of other bodies who have left no more mark on the earth than a leaf leaves on the storm. That must be the plan of the Creator, for it is certainly the way of all flesh.

Cancer makes us think about death, doesn't it? Even if we have every confidence that we shall recover, be cured, be saved from this particular hit man sent by the cancer Mafia, we are reminded that some day we shall die. For many of us, cancer will be the cause of death. Most of us still, the first time we hear that word applied to us, immediately think of death.

I have the normal fears of death and dying, but they are not the reason for this leap forward to grief that I am experiencing now. You see, I, and I alone, in this particular brain and body, have certain memories, specific hopes, particular clusters of relationships, my own peculiar way of seeing the world. When I am gone, the whole universe of my experience is gone. Not only are my language and my knowledge and my relationships gone, but all the effort I put into learning to read and understand and be a friend is also no more. Who else knows how it feels to be twenty years old and hear Helen say for the first time, "I love you"? Who else remembers what it was like to be the first McFarland or Pond to receive a college diploma? Who else ever dreamed that he hit a home run to win the World Series the same day his twelve-volume *History of the World* was published?

God must be crazy to be so profligate, developing each human being, body and soul, so uniquely and completely .. and then letting all that go in death! How stupid. How inefficient. Think of all that waste, all the starting over, all that's lost each time this happens. Why, you'd think the world is infinite, that space goes on forever, that God has all the time in the world, acting that way!

Is God simply experimenting with us, trying one after another until one of us finally gets it right? If one of us does finally get it right, will everyone from then on be exactly like that one, will she or he be the pattern for all to come?

I suspect not. I think God has something else in mind. (You may not want to use the word "God" here, and that is perfectly okay, of course; substitute your own word, because it's the one you've been given in your uniqueness to use.) I am convinced, by faith but also by reason, that God is telling us something by acting in this crazy way. I think we're being told that Love is at the heart of everything—space and time and life—and that Love is boundless, infinite, without measure. It does not need to be conserved or reused. There is enough to go around, enough that each individual can have his or her uniqueness.

Workers in the field of addictions tell us that at the heart of any addiction is the belief that love is limited, that there isn't enough to go around, that it has to be hoarded. When one feels left out from limited love is when addictions develop, to try to fill the empty spaces.

Death, strangely, is God's way of saying it isn't so, of letting us know that Love has no limits, that there is so much Love to go around that each of us can have a unique life in this world and pass on without a trace of us remaining and the level of love isn't lowered even a little bit.

> *Now that I have cancer, I grieve already for*
> *the loss my death will bring to the world,*
> *for I am unique; no one can replace me.*
> *But that uniqueness is also a word of Love.*
> *There is great sadness in the thought of my*
> *uniqueness passing from the scene, but there*
> *is great hope in the limitlessness of Love.*

... I get termination notices.

I COULDN'T BELIEVE IT! I ordered a trial subscription to a cancer journal for patients. When it ran out, they sent me a *termination* notice! Big black letters. Black edges around the envelope.

I wrote them. "Don't you know what a 'termination notice' means to a cancer patient?" I asked. "Your whole magazine is for patients; how could you be so insensitive?" I never heard back from them. I suppose they figured it wasn't worth it; I'd probably be terminated soon, anyway.

I don't want to get a termination notice. I want to live, forever. I want everything to go on just the way it is (except for the nausea).

If I get terminated, I'll never get to be an old man, and I was so looking forward to being an old man. Not just any old man. I want to be an irascible old curmudgeon. (My wife, of course, says that I don't have to worry; I've already made it.)

You can get away with so much when you're old that you can't when you're younger. You can get discounts, too.

I've looked like an old man for a long time. I went bald and gray early. My unruly white beard makes me resemble Santa enough that strange little children ask me for toys. I've looked like I was seventy-five since I was forty-five. There's an advantage to that. If I ever do get old, people will say, "You know, he hasn't aged a bit." Then they'll think I "look good for my age."

When I was forty-seven, I ran into a supermarket one

day to get a can of dog food for Waggs, even though she favors people food. It was a big mistake. I had forgotten it was senior citizen day. I was trying to rush to the dog-food aisle and out again, but there was a "comparison" convention taking place in the store.

"I can remember when this dog food can was only forty-nine cents," someone would say.

A voice would come from over in the hot-cereal section. "That's nothing; I remember when it was only thirty-nine cents."

It was like an auction. "Thirty-four. Twenty-nine. Twenty-five. Twenty-two? Anyone for twenty-two? Twenty-five once . . ."

I grabbed a can of Cycle Old Dog and ran to the checkout lane. A young woman who couldn't have been more than a year out of high school was running the items through the scanner.

"That'll be fifty-six, with the discount."

"What discount?" I asked, assuming there must be a "good looks" discount or "great body" discount.

"Why, it's senior citizens' day," she replied. "You get the senior citizens' discount, don't you?"

I wanted to shout, "How old do you think I am?" I decided against it, though. I was afraid she might tell me.

You know what I do now? If they give me the discount without asking if I'm eligible, I take it. I figure it's compensation for pain and suffering. I also figure it's one way I can get to be an irascible old curmudgeon, regardless of how long I live.

I guess I objected to getting the discount because it was a little termination notice, a way of saying someone thinks I'm a day closer to death. But you know, they're right. I am.

Each of us is, regardless of the state of our health. Every day is a termination notice.

That makes me rethink this whole notion. If each day is a termination notice, then I do want to keep on getting them.

I've spent my life making memories for other people. When I'm finally terminated, I want folks to fill the gap of my presence with those memories. In the meantime, I'll just keep on making memories.

Now that I have cancer,
I'm glad for every day and every notice.

WHEN "YOU'RE THE DOCTOR"

. . . *I'm the doctor.*

M Y SURGEON FORGOT I was in the hospital! (You can read the full story of this in the meditation on remembering where you are.) Flat out thought I'd gone home, so he didn't come in for three days, until I had the nurse call him up to find out where he was. I'm not sure why he thought I was gone, since he hadn't dismissed me. Just busy, I guess.

I was busy, too, however—busy getting my five tubes unhooked every morning at five A.M. so I could stagger on to the scales to be reminded I couldn't eat, busy drinking that grape juice they strain through nuclear waste to give it that tangy taste, and then busy throwing up in that little curved pan, busy lying around waiting for the doctor to come in to take care of me.

Then an oncologist I'd never met and didn't know from a flea-bottomist came in, right after I was weighed, and told me I had "it." *"It?"* "Cancer, of course. I'll call the National Cancer Institute to see if there's any adjuvant therapy, but I doubt it." *"Adjuvant? What does that mean?"* "You've got a 70 percent chance of recurrence in one to two years." *"Cancer? Adjuvant? What are you going to do about it?"* But he was already gone. . . .

The surgeon forgot about me. The oncologist said there wasn't anything to do about it and that I'd be dead in a year or two.

I went to a different oncologist at another hospital. He was recommended by a friend.

"Yes," he said, "there is a therapy for you, twelve months

of chemotherapy that will make you sick as a dog. (He likes to talk that medical jargon—you are either "sick as a dog" or "healthy as a horse.") If you're going to do it, though, we have to start today. Go out in the waiting room and talk it over with your wife."

So I sat there, bent over from the surgery, holding hands with Helen in the waiting room, a room full of thirty sick and sympathetic-looking patients, knowing I had one choice to make, that I had to make it now. She squeezed my hand and said, "For what it's worth, I know what I would do if it were my body. . . ."

If it were my body? But it wasn't *my* body! I just live in it. It's the doctors' job to take care of my body, to make it well, isn't it? But my doctor forgot me . . . and said there wasn't any therapy for me . . . and told me to take my time but do it now.

It *is* my body! It's *my* job to take care of it! *I'm* the doctor!

My surgeon is an excellent knife-wielder. My second oncologist is an excellent researcher and diagnostician and chemo-pusher. But I'm the doctor, the only one finally who has the responsibility for my body, for my life.

One thing the medical researchers have learned is that a patient deteriorates rapidly at the moment of diagnosis, the moment you get that news, that you first hear that word. It is important for the physician to tell the patient what the diagnosis is in a way that challenges but that does not hurt the possibility of recovery.

For at least two weeks after I was told I had cancer, told early in the morning by a stranger with none of my loved ones present, told that my best chance was 30 percent, I simply prepared to die. Then a lot of people who love me began to tell me, without ever saying it in so many words, "You make the diagnosis. You don't have to live with what anyone else has said, and you don't have to die with it. You're responsible for your own life. We trust you to be the doctor."

I was always the type who said to the man or woman in the white coat, with the stethoscope around the neck, "You're the doctor." We say that, don't we? If the mechanic tells us we need a new water pump, we reply, "You're the doctor." If a plumber says we need a new faucet, we say, "You're the doctor." That very phrase is part of our culture. It says that we are going to turn it over to the expert, to the "doctor" for that particular field.

Well, when it comes to me, I'm the doctor, I'm the expert, I'm the one who has to make the decisions. I need the oncologists and the radiologists and the nurses and the pharmacists, but they are *my* assistants, not the other way around. Perhaps the best thing my physician could have done for me was to forget I was in the hospital.

Now that I have cancer, I'm the doctor!

... I create my own life.

I'M THE ONLY ONE WHO HAS CONTROL of how I interpret events. I can see any occasion of my life as a "bummer" or as an opportunity. It will be however I see it, because there is no outside, objective standard by which to judge.

For instance, no one or nothing else can make me angry. Someone else might do something I don't like or that I think is unfair, but I'm the one who decides if I'll be angry. Your boss might fire you, your husband might leave you, your child might disappoint you, but you are the one who creates your life, not the boss or husband or child.

That's always been true, of course, but I didn't really understand it before.

Viktor Frankl, the psychiatrist, was a prisoner in a Nazi death camp during World War II. His wife was killed there. From that experience, he says he learned that there is one freedom no one can ever take away from you, the freedom to decide how you will react to the circumstances around you. Cancer is my death-camp experience.

That makes me rethink the story of Job. Job was a good man, a blameless man. Every imaginable evil happened to Job, just so God could prove Job's faithfulness to the devil. His friends kept saying, "There must have been something you did to bring this on yourself." Job consistently protested his innocence, and he asked God for an explanation. "How come me? What did I do?" He didn't get an answer. All God said, in effect, was: "If I told you, you wouldn't understand, and I'm not going to tell you, anyhow." Job never got an explanation. He could have "cursed God and died," as his friends advised, and surely he would have been justified in doing so. But he was faithful. In the face of his loss of wealth and family, in the face of his friends' sarcasm, in the face of God's arrogant silence, Job made his own decision how he would react. He created his own life.

How I react to cancer makes all the difference. It's what I believe, what I imagine, the attitude I take, that decides whether I shall live or die. That may be true even in a physical sense, because it's often been proved that a tree's fruit is consistent. A healthy attitude makes for a healthy body. I'm speaking not just of the body, however, as important as it is, but of the spirit, where the real decisions are made, where the real life is created.

Cancer has made me see things in my life that need to be corrected. My defensiveness, for instance. In any situation—a conversation or meeting or transaction at a store—my first reaction is defensive. I expect to be criticized. I spend long hours anticipating every complaint anyone could make and then think up every possible rebuttal. This is called "awfulizing," imagining the most awful situation conceivable. Of course, such detraction hardly ever happens, and if someone does find fault, it's usually not a charge I had considered anyway! Consequently very few people have any idea how negative and self-protective I am.

I've been defensive as long as I can remember, but I had gotten used to it. I just accepted it as part of life. Suddenly I had to ask myself, "If I have only a year or two to live, do I want to spend it being defensive?" The answer is "No, because it's not worth it, and because it won't help me get well." I'm taking charge. I'm deciding how I'll spend my mind. I'm creating my own life.

One of the marks of a long-term survivor is following a personal health plan that you think will have good results. I know there's no simple route to being well, no easy program to follow. Getting well, getting whole, comes from a whole series of small decisions. Together, though, they make up the one big decision, the choice to create your own life. When you've made that choice, you're already healed, even if your body doesn't know it.

Now that I have cancer, I create my own life.

. . . I wonder why I got it.

D O I HAVE SOME SECRET DEATH WISH? Is that why, even now, I try to ignore it, try to go back to my old, fragmented ways of living?

They say cancer often develops in response to a loss, especially in the previous year or two. But I can't think of any great loss that's come my way. A little loss of energy, maybe. Some loss of ambition. My hair's been misplaced for a long time. Besides, I don't think those are the kinds of losses the books are talking about. They mean the loss of a loved one, or a job, or a reason to live.

I've lived a wholesome lifestyle for years—eaten a healthy diet, loved and been loved, done meaningful work, gotten plenty of exercise. So why did this cancer choose this year to make its invasion?

Of course, I could claim that this cancer doesn't have anything to do with my past lifestyle at all. It's just happenstance, or fate.

A few years ago, my eighteen- and nineteen-year-old nephews were killed together in an auto crash, along with two of their friends. The night of the visitation at the funeral home, the only remaining brother of one of the other dead boys took the family car out and managed to drive recklessly enough that he turned it over and broke his leg.

"How could you do that?" I asked him. "Your brother is lying dead in the funeral home. You are your parents' only living child. Don't you have any concern, at least, for them?"

94

He shrugged his shoulders. "I've got no control over it," he said. "When it's my time to go, I'll have to go."

No control over it, he said. The speed, the quick cornering, not wearing a seat belt, not stopping at red lights—those didn't have anything to do with whether he lived or died!

There's something appealing about that, isn't there? Life is just out of my control. I'm only the helpless subject of outside forces, whether they're the cigarettes that force themselves into my mouth or pesticides on the apricots or the chemicals the "Jungle Growth" Company spreads on my neighbor's lawn. I have nothing to do with it, so I can't be blamed.

We live in a "no-fault" time, don't we? No-fault divorce, no-fault car insurance, no-fault everything. We have such a hard time handling guilt that we just legislate it out of existence . . . until it comes in the back door under an assumed name. I want "no-fault" cancer.

The problem with that is that if I can't find what I did to contribute to my cancer, then I can't reverse that process to contribute to my cure. If I've got no fault, I've got no solution.

Sure, I can say "outside" forces caused it, so I can use outside forces like chemotherapy and radiation to cure it. I just happen to be the man in the middle.

There's a way in which that is true. I have no doubt that outside forces helped bring about my cancer. I'm extremely grateful for the outside force of my chemotherapy. I can't, however, just leave it at that.

I have to examine, at least, what I contributed, with the way I eat or the way I think, so I can change the way I eat and the way I think. I don't want to leave anything to chance. I want to have a part in getting well. I'm not just a battleground for warring armies. I'm one of the generals.

So, why did I get it, especially now? I'm not sure yet, but I thank God for the chance to wonder about it . . . and to work at it. . . .

. . . *I have to pay* . . .

PAY THE PRICE FOR MY OWN LIFE.
The mother of a friend died. He felt his father should move into a nursing home, but the father refused. He insisted on staying in his own home. Each weekend, my friend went to his father's town, took him shopping, did the laundry, got his medicines.

After ten years, close to his death, the father said, "See, you didn't think it would work out for me to stay alone, but I've done just fine."

Shaking his head, my friend said, "He thought he had done just fine, but I was the one who didn't have a weekend for ten years. I paid the price for his lifestyle."

Who pays the price for you?

There's a great irony about price paying. The more each of us pays the price for his or her own life, the closer we are drawn together. The more each of us walks alone, the closer we walk shoulder-to-shoulder in the travels and travails of life.

Right now I'm more at one with others than I have ever been, but I'm also more alone than I've ever been.

I felt that especially in the hospital. My wife, my children, my friends, the nurses—they all did everything they could for me, but they couldn't move my bowels. They couldn't stand up and urinate for me. They could walk with me down the hall, but they couldn't take my particular, puny steps. They couldn't drink that awful, chemical-tasting grape juice for me, and I'm glad they didn't have to! It was a strange, lonesome journey, and I had to walk it by myself.

You are not real until you pay the price for your own life. Walking that lonely valley is how you pay that price. You have to take responsibility for yourself, for your own health and wholeness, even though you cannot always effect a cure for your illness any more than the doctors and nurses can.

Well, let me not talk for you. I can't say, "*You* must take responsibility. . . ." I can only say, "*I* must take responsibility for my own life." I must make the footprints of my particular journey. I can't walk yours. You can't walk mine.

There's another feeling, however, along with the aloneness. The oneness.

How is it that we are so much in oneness when each of us walks finally alone? Somehow we are never more united than when each of us is paying the price for his or her own life. I don't quite understand this, but I know it to be true.

Who pays the price for your life, for your lifestyle? We so often say to husband or wife or children or parents or friends or neighbors, "You pay. You pay for me. I can't pay. I have nothing with which to pay. You pay the price for me." We have a thousand ways to make them pay. When, however, each of us says, "I'll pay my own way; I'll take the responsibility for me," then we have turned one another loose for love.

We walk alone, but as we do, we walk together. Alone, together, we walk in the courage of freedom and love.

> *Now that I have cancer,*
> *I have to pay the price for my own life.*

WHEN IT'S TIME TO GIVE THANKS

. . . I never have a bad day.

I HAVE NAUSEATED DAYS and frightened days. Tired days and hurting days. Long days and short days. Silent days and alone days. Mouth-sore days and swollen-hand days. Bald days and diarrhea days. Rainy days and sunny days. Cold days and warm days. But no bad days.

Every day with cancer is like a month without it. Cancer has a way of getting your attention. I sometimes say that I lived more in the first month after I found out I had cancer than I did in the previous fifty-three years. It's not that the previous fifty-three were bad years. Some elephant-sized things happened for me in those years. I got married. I fathered and helped raise my children. I made lifelong friends. I worked for good causes. Those years, however, went by in a blur.

My father-in-law, Earl "Tank" Karr, used to say that after age forty, the days went by at propeller speed. Suddenly you were old, and you didn't know what had become of the years.

Every cancer moment is intense. It makes you focus.

Sometimes it's the focus that the eyes of a rabbit fix on a fox, the focus of fear, the bunching of the muscles to run.

Sometimes, though, it's a focus of longing, of feeling the beauty of life so clearly that you can express it only in words of hyperbole: "Behold, you are beautiful, my love! Your eyes are doves behind your veil. Your hair is like a flock of goats, moving down the slopes of Gilead. . . . Your cheeks are like halves of a pomegranate . . ." (Song of

Solomon, chapter 4). Any woman (or man) today would think you'd slipped a gear if you tried that for romance! Solomon knew, however, that even though some feelings are so strong they can't be put into words, you have to try anyway. Thus you have to make it clear that the words you use express the depth of your emotion even though they don't make "sense." Indeed, if they made sense they would only bob upon the surface, not go down deep.

Cancer brings up that sort of emotion about life, and thus that inability to say in so many words what life means. When I say "I don't have a bad day," anyone outside of cancer doesn't understand. They look at me, with my puffy lips and my running eyes and my behind so sore I can't sit down, and they say, without words, "It looks bad enough to me."

Of course it's a bad day, but it's *my* day. Every moment is full. There is no time that is idle. Each moment may be filled with fear or nausea or pain, but it is full! That's why it's not a "bad" moment, or a "bad" day.

There's a story about a man who offered a $10,000 reward for the return of his wife's pet cat. His friends were astounded, for they knew that he loathed and despised that cat.

"Why are you offering so much for that cat's return when you hate it so much?" they asked.

"Ah," he said with a wink, "when you know what you know, you can afford to be extravagant."

For he knew that he had already drowned and buried his wife's pet cat!

When you know what you know, you can afford to be extravagant with each moment, living it to the fullest, putting everything you have into that one point in time, because that's all there is. I know what I know—that it is cancer that is weak and I who am strong. There's no need to hold back, to save anything for what will come, because all that might come is already here. This is the day that is, my day.

Now that I have cancer, I never have a bad day.

. . . I rejoice in my miseries.

I DON'T MEAN IN SPITE OF MY MISERIES; I mean *in* my miseries.

It is because of my miseries that I have been contacted by so many old friends and met so many new ones. It is because of my miseries that I have learned so much about myself, and about what is important in life. It is because of my miseries that I feel I have lived more in a few months of cancer time than I did in fifty years of "ordinary" time. It is because of my miseries that I feel connected to Love in ways I never dreamed of before.

I'm thankful for pain and side effects and disruptions in my careful schedules and new limits that hedge me in. They all sing to me a song of life. They are reminders of how precious life is.

I wrote a poem about this experience, this strange and paradoxical feeling of being thankful in misery.

PAIN

And finally, now, unwanted friend,
we die together, not alone . . .
as we have lived.
You are the only one who walks
the final step with me,
the step they claim we take,
at last, alone.
Until I go, you stay.
When I go, you must.
As long as you are with me,

I remain.
So no brash miracles for me,
to snatch you far away.
Without you, I am gone.
As you grow stronger,
I grow weak.
(Funny, that we call the weakness
growth.)
Only together do we knit the whole.
Stay awhile, if you will,
for I shall miss you.
Even you, I shall miss.

I'm not romantic about pain. Sometimes it is so bad, so overpowering. It engulfs you and makes anything else, especially rejoicing, impossible. But even pain can't remain forever. And yes, I'll miss even it, because it is a reminder that I am yet alive.

There's a story about a young man who returned home after several years in military service. He was inquiring about what had happened to various people in the old neighborhood while he was away.

"Is old man Brown alive yet?" he asked.

"No, not yet," came the reply.

Life isn't automatic just because our bodies are functioning and unbroken. We don't live from birth to death but from tomb to tomb, first the tomb of the womb and then the tomb that marks the end of our particular time span on this earth. Beyond each of those tombs is the possibility of life or death.

You're not alive until you can feel the pain. Is old McFarland alive yet? Now that I have cancer, I am.

Now that I have cancer, I rejoice in my miseries.

. . . I wear my "glasses."

THEY'RE REALLY "PLASTICS," and I always wear them, of course. At least I do if I want to read. I can see everything else just fine without them. But not words.

I bring the book up close, right against my nose, which my younger daughter has always assured me looks remarkably like a strawberry. Just a blur—the words, not my nose. I rattle and shake the newspaper until it is halfway across the room, or at least as far as my thirty-four-inch sleeve will push it. No luck—black and white, but not "read all over."

Then I slip my remarkably stylish smoke-gray bifocals up onto my strawberry and over my ears and "Voilà!" and "Eureka!" and all those other words that mean "Hallelujah!" I can see! Words! Not just a smudge of ink, but words. . . .

Talk about your miracles. I slip in front of my misty blues a thin film of plastic, and immediately I'm in touch with the world—Moses and Jesus and Rousseau and old Bill Shakespeare and Tom Jefferson and Edna Ferber and Dave Barry.

Cancer's like that, isn't it? It's a lens slipped down in front of our eyes. Suddenly there's a whole new world to see. It's a strange new world, frightening in its strangeness, but there's a certain clarity, a point of focus, in all that newness.

Ray Bradbury, in *The Martian Chronicles*, has a scene set in Independence, Missouri, the jumping-off point for the old wagon trains heading west. In his book, way into the future, it is the jumping-off point for people who are going off to live in space. A young woman has gone there, to catch the next spaceship to Mars, to join her fiancé there. She will live the rest of her life with him on an alien planet, a place she has never seen.

She is terrified. She doesn't know if she can go through with it. She calls him on the space telephone and pours out all her fears and doubts. He replies, but most of what he says is blanked out by static. The space telephone is not perfected, so they cannot talk back and forth. It is just her speech and then his speech and the conversation is over.

She doesn't really know what he said. From within the garble and static, she is able to pick out only one word. In his voice, she hears the word *love*. On the strength of that one word, the next day she launches herself into space and a new life.

In all the garble of words like *levamisole* and *5-FU* and *metastasize* and *PNI* there is still a word of focus. It's always been there, but maybe we weren't wearing the right glasses to be able to see it. Cancer is a great gift if it provides the lens of love.

It's a whole new world, as scary as the thought of living on Mars, but as we see the word of Love, we can take the step and go. . . .

Now that I have cancer, I wear my "glasses."

. . . *I'm thankful for the cancer.*

THE IDEA SORT OF SEEPED INTO ME. No thunder-claps or lightning bolts, just a quiet awareness. I was walking, slowly, a half block farther than I'd been since the surgery. Enough of the nippy April morning remained that the sun's spring-violet light still slanted and winked at me through first-bud branches. I began to hurt, to step even slower, to worry about whether I could get home, to won-der if I knew someone along the way who would give me a ride. It wasn't much of a context for giving thanks.

That's how it came, though, and when. I began to talk to myself, to urge myself on. Then I began to pray, to talk to God, to ask for help, for strength, just enough power and courage to push me three blocks home. I heard me say it—overheard, actually, as though it were a different person speaking: "I'm thankful for the cancer."

I guess it *was* a different person who said it.

What happens in life is that we get used to the unlovely parts. It's like having season tickets in the corner of the sta-dium for the football games. There's one section of the field you never see, but you get used to it, so used to your partial view that you don't even ask for better seats next year.

Or consider the "floaters" in front of our eyes. They ob-scure our vision, but most of the time, we're not even aware of them. They're always there. In fact, we don't want to no-tice them too much, for when we do, they bother us all the more.

We go through life working and playing, but not really paying attention. Cancer gets your attention. The threat of death is part of it. Cancer is a fatal disease, unless . . . unless you do something about it. We don't have the option of doing nothing and continuing to live. So we have to choose—will I face it, will I fight it, or will I just die? If I strike back, there's a chance I'll have more life in this body, but there's no guarantee.

One way or the other I have to face the fact, *really* face it, that my days are limited. What will I do with them?

In days gone by, when a young man was trying to capture the affections of a young woman, it was said that he was "paying attention to her." It's still a good phrase. When someone is romantically interested in another, she or he pays attention to that person and tries to attract attention in return. The problem is that so often after we have been successful, and nabbed the object of our interest, then we *stop* paying attention.

I once knew a married couple who lived in separate wings of their house. They drove separate cars and went to different movies. There didn't seem to be animosity between them, but they just didn't pay attention to each other. One day I asked the woman why she had married the man, since they seemed to have so little in common.

"Well," she said, "he just kept after me, and the only way I knew to get rid of him was to marry him."

It's easy enough to do that with life, to get rid of it by marrying it. Then we can go our separate way, live in the far room, stop paying attention.

Cancer forces us to look at life again, to notice the part of the playing field we can't see. It gives us the opportunity to look at all the unlovely things about ourselves that we've gotten so used to that we do nothing about them. It gives us a chance to get our lives into shape.

I suspect folks get tired of hearing me say this, but I'll try it again anyway: I think I've lived more in the few months since I got cancer than I did in all the years before. I'm more aware of life, have better focus, experience each moment. I'm paying attention, and that lets me separate the wheat from the chaff.

Now that I have cancer, I'm thankful.

. . . I'm vulnerable . . .

AND I WANT TO TAKE ADVANTAGE of that vulnerability. I want to keep on being the new me.

Maybe I'll slide back with time. Perhaps my footprints on the sands of time won't be so crisp, so nicely edged, but instead will show that crumbling pattern of the one who slips back with each step almost as far as he strides. Maybe I'll go back to shaking hands instead of hugging. Maybe I'll fall back to choking off the tears instead of letting them flow. Maybe I'll want to be "strong" again instead of open.

I don't want to backslide. I don't want to wall off instead of weep out, but I know it can happen. When my chemotherapy is over, and the cards and letters stop, and I have passed my five year test and can eat colored food again, what happens if I become the old, "strong" me again?

"Strong" isn't bad. It isn't everything, either.

I like the new me, who weeps to see the little neighbor girl ride her bright, pink bike, just because a healthy child in motion is such a beautiful sight.

I like the me who surprises men in gray suits with a big hug. It's a wonderful sight, two men in pinstripes, trying to figure out what to do with their briefcases while they attempt a hug—good laughter therapy if nothing else!

I like the me who talks to trees to let them know how well they are doing and how good they are looking.

I like the me who sings prayers, and laughs at silliness, and hopes all the time, without even knowing it, because it's so much a part of me.

I like the me who wakes up in the morning feeling joyful that there is so much to do instead of burdened because there is so much to do.

I like the me who welcomes pain as a friend because it reminds me that I am alive.

I like the me who isn't bothered by the chaos of my desk but covers it over with the sure knowledge of what is important and what is not.

I like the me who trusts the Spirit more than the calendar and date books and lists and planners.

I've always had the cool, silent, determined courage of strength. Now I have the warm, bubbling, winging courage of weakness as well.

So I pray: "Let me grow, in both health and illness, into the new me. Let me be worthy of the new me. Let me be thankful for the old me—for the old me was a gift, too—but keep me vulnerable. Let every part of me move toward the whole me."

Now that I have cancer,
I'm vulnerable . . . and scared . . . and glad.

. . . I have permission to pay attention to my self.

I T SEEMS THAT SOME FOLKS pay attention to nothing else. Their lives are bordered on the north, south, east, and west by . . . self . . . and that's all. They remind me of the man who prayed thus: "Bless me and my wife, our son, John, and his wife; us four and no more. Amen."

Most of us who get cancer, though, aren't like that. We're "pretty good people." We work hard. We feel guilty if we don't get things done. We blame ourselves if things go wrong. We feel that we have to make the world a better place. We're embarrassed if we're not "making a difference." For people like us, any attention at all to our selves is "selfishness."

Besides, we really are busy. We have jobs and families and friends and organizations. The whole world conspires to jam us in traffic and never to be there when we telephone and to get in line in front of us in the supermarket. There's just no time for self! We've got cars that are past their oil change mileage and toilets that are fighting back and children who are tugging at our legs and . . . Even in those spare moments when we look wistfully toward the unread books and recall the times we prayed or meditated, there's no time to follow up.

So we've become machines instead of people, robots rather than persons, lists instead of lovers, date books rather than selves.

Now, however, there's a clearing in the forest. It's burnt

over harshly, down to the stubble, but it's still a clearing. It gives me a chance to see with a wider view, a vision of the sky.

Now it's okay for me to take the time to visualize, to pray, to read, to nap, to sit, to stare, to meditate . . . to be.

A man dies and we hear someone ask, "What was he worth?" "Oh, probably half a million," someone answers. Half a million what? Embraces? Prayers? Loves? Kindnesses? Sunsets? Bird songs? Walks? Meals with friends? "Of course not! Half a million *dollars!*" Is that all someone is worth? Dollars? If it's dollars, then it doesn't make any difference whether it's five or five billion. The same is true with all the other events and activities by which we usually measure worth. Did she make vice president? So what? Was he the star? Big deal. A forty-year pin? Big whoop!

It's not what you *do* but what you *are!* That's where this business of self comes in. My life has meaning not because I'm acceptable, but because I'm accepted, not because I'm lovable, but because I'm loved. I'm a part of Life, a child of God. I *am!* Whether in this life or some other life, I *am.* I'm not a statistical summary—worked thirty years, married once, fathered two, made some bucks, watched some TV.

So now that I have cancer, it's okay just to be. Somehow I have permission from myself and the rest of the world to concentrate on this self, in order to get well. In the process, I have a chance not just to get cured, but to get whole, to be who I'm meant to be.

Now that I have cancer,
I have permission to pay attention to my self.

. . . *I live in shared space.*

I SIT IN THIS SHARED SPACE, in the waiting room of the cancer center, with people I have never seen before and may never see again. As I read their faces, though, I know we'll be forever in the same space, together.

Some of these faces simply stare into the middle distance, as though the space is empty. Some have eyes that I can see, but I know that they are staring into inner space. I can tell which is which, but I'm not sure just how I know the difference.

An old lady is eating a donut. A large plastic bag, cracked with age and cheapness, sits on the floor beside her chair; it is full of flowers. Her hair is pinned to her head with barrettes, but it's escaping in little wisps of gray—the color of memory. She's stuck into an ancient green pantsuit, twenty years out of fashion. Her face sags with an infinite sadness. One eye is clouded, as though it remembers only milkweed, but remembers it well. The donut looks very small in her large and rough hands. They look like hands that have done the work they had to do. Because of that, they are beautiful.

It is clear that the donut is the highlight of her day. She takes tiny bites; it lasts longer that way. She holds each wee bite in her mouth, not chewing, letting it dissolve in a slow mirth upon her tongue. Every bite is both a memory and a hope.

The tall, handsome man across from her uncoils and saunters to the donut table. He plucks one casually, rolls back to his seat. He looks like Rock Hudson doing a John

Wayne imitation. He's draped in a new tweed Western suit, above shiny, two-tone cowboy boots. A bolo tie graces the front of his striped shirt. His fourteen-dollar haircut insists that each strand keep the peace. His cowboy hat sits importantly in a place of honor in the chair next to him, trying to call attention away from the body he is trying to hide. He eats the donut as though he has no place to go, no past, and no future down inside him.

The man and woman with the white hair look alike. Their glasses, their clothes, their hairstyles, the way they cross their legs, even the shapes of their bodies, match. They have been together for a long time. They share a donut, passing it back and forth, each taking a precise bite, no larger or smaller than the other. If I could see them kiss, I would see the lines of their cheeks match, flow together, groove into each other, so I could not tell where one begins and the other ends.

We share this room, this box of donuts, this space, although not by choice. This is a space of both despair and hope, fear and faith, anxiety and love. It is our space, together. I'm glad we share the space and the donuts and the hope.

I wonder what the other faces here read when they look toward me. Will they tell at the dinner table about the strange bald man who watched and wrote? Do they notice that I cut my donut in half, eat one side, then the other? Do they read that as a man divided, not whole? If so, they are right. But they also see a man whose eyes are wet with tears of solidarity, as he watches the other donut eaters in this shared space. Because of that, next time they'll see a man without a knife.

Now that I have cancer, I live in shared space.

WHEN IT'S TIME FOR NEW THINKING

... *It's a touching time.*

MY FRIEND BILL came to see me, a week after I was out of the hospital. He drove a hundred miles each way to spend an hour with me. We've been friends through almost thirty years. Between us we've had three wives and seven children. We don't see each other often, but we don't need to; our friendship is always still there. Bill's first wife left him ten years ago. Just told him one day she was leaving. No previous symptoms, even in retrospect. Just like my cancer. We share that kind of surprised grieving—he in his first marriage, me in my body.

When he was ready to leave, he sat on the sofa beside me and put his arm around me. I held on to his leg, like a little boy might wrap his arm around a father's knee. We prayed together. He told me he loved me. I tried to tell him I loved him, too, but I couldn't get it out. I believe he understood, though. Other than shaking hands, I think that's the first time we've touched, in thirty years.

Now that I have cancer, there seems to be an unspoken word of permission for people to touch me, for me to touch them. It's funny, that a broken body should somehow be more touchable than one that's "whole." Or am I more touchable because my spirit is broken? "The sacrifice acceptable to God is a broken spirit; a broken and a contrite heart, O God, you will not despise" (Psalm 51:17). It is interesting that in all the stories of Jesus, there is only one instance of anyone touching him while he was alive in the body. He, of course, touched many—a leper, a hand to raise Simon's mother-in-law or Jairus's daughter up from beds of illness and death, deaf ears, blind eyes, the feet of the disciples, children. The woman with the hemorrhage only reached as far as the hem of his robe. The woman who broke the alabaster jar of ointment on his feet wiped it off with her hair—no touch. The only time anyone reached out to touch Jesus was to betray him, Judas with a kiss, the authorities of his own faith and people with a slap.

Maybe that's why "doubting" Thomas insisted on his famous touch-and-feel session after the crucifixion. Perhaps he was really "knowing" Thomas. Since no one had touched Jesus while he was alive, Thomas knew the real proof of the resurrection was that he could be touched, his body was broken. It's only after the breaking of crucifixion that resurrection, the touching time, comes.

Somehow we seem able to touch one another in our brokenness in ways we never can in wholeness. God likes to use broken things—broken bread, broken ointment jars, broken bodies, even relationships broken with a kiss.

> *My body and my spirit have been broken by cancer.*
> *That means I can touch and be touched.*
> *I'm thankful for the cancer.*

. . . I listen to myself.

I LISTEN TO THE WORLD AROUND ME, but I also listen to the world inside me. I listen to myself.

Most of us go through life without listening to ourselves, our own bodies and spirits. Thus we never know what we need, so we never get what we need.

Many of us are taught early on to be quiet about our own needs. You'd think that being quiet would lead to good listening, but it doesn't. It seems to work the other way around. The quieter we become, the harder it is to hear.

Sometimes our parents don't respond to our cries as infants, don't hold us, don't let us feel their love. We learn that there is no point in asking, so we "shut up," quite completely. We shut ourselves up in cells of silence. Often we are rewarded for our quiet, are called "good" girls and boys because we shut ourselves up. We become proud that we never tell anyone what we need. We are silent, and we equate that with strength. We stop listening to the night cries of our souls because we'll never tell anyone what we hear anyway.

Others of us silence ourselves with our own voices. We talk incessantly, tell anyone about our problems, whine constantly, curse the day we were born and every other day as well. We prattle on just to hear our own sounds, because they remind us that we still exist. Those around us get tired and stop listening. We get bored, too, and quit listening to ourselves. We resemble Dylan Thomas's famous remark: "Someone is boring me. I think it's me." After all, we've heard it hundreds of times.

Our credo is found in a conversation you can hear any day in any small town post office:

"How ya doin'?"

"Can't complain."

"Wouldn't do any good, anyhow."

Since it won't do any good, we don't bother to learn what there is to complain about, to listen to learn what our own needs are.

Now, though, I listen. Not so I can complain to others, or even to myself, but so I know who I am, so I can take control of my own life rather than leaving me shut up in some cell of silence. I have to know what I need, even if no one else does, because I am the one who has responsibility for taking care of this self. If I don't accept that responsibility, I'll have no self to be responsible for anything else.

"Fool, said I, you do not know / Silence like a cancer grows." Those are lines from Simon and Garfunkle's hit song "The Sounds of Silence." Silence grows like a cancer, and cancer grows in the silence. Not the silence of no sound, but the silence of no listening. If we don't listen to ourselves, we can't listen to others, either.

There's a story about a piece of marble in Florence, Italy. All the sculptors rejected it, because it was so ugly. Then Michelangelo came along one day and saw David trying to get out of it. Thus came one of the greatest pieces of art of all time. I suspect that Michelangelo listened not only to the cries of David, calling for freedom from the marble, but that he listened to himself as well.

I heard of an old man whose family asked him, in disgust, why he talked to himself all the time. "Why, because I like to hear what I have to say," he replied. It's a pretty good reason, and a pretty good thing to do.

I certainly haven't given up on listening to my doctors and my friends and my family. But I listen to myself as well. My body and my spirit are telling me what I need. It's really okay to trust what I hear.

Now that I have cancer, I listen to myself.

. . . *I go slow* . . .

EVER SO SLOW. (I know it's not grammatical, but I like the sound of it, don't you?) Going slow is a luxury in our world. It's also a gift from cancer.

I've aged twenty years in five months. I hope to get twenty years younger in another eight months, when my chemo is over, but in the meantime, I'm a much older, and slower, guy.

That has some advantages. I'm more empathetic with older people than I used to be. I come up behind some slow mover in the oatmeal aisle and I don't dash around her as I used to, with a huff and a puff, showing off my young legs and eager lungs. So what if she has the aisle blocked with a prairie schooner that contains two small plain yogurts and a carrot? It's important to stand there and read all the labels, to see how many grams of fat lurk in each brand. Now I might even linger a bit and point out to her that I like "Uncle Ted's" in the plain white box best, because it has fewer preservatives than "Nature's Normal All Natural," the one with the eight-color picture of a golden sun rising over a field of herbicides. (You just can't trust cereal box pictures, unless the picture is of Michael Jordan, of course.)

One reason I don't hurry around the other shoppers, I must admit, is that I can't. When you are aging a year per day, you slow down in a hurry. Besides that, my immune system is depressed by the chemotherapy, and I'm on a blood thinner because of the Groshong catheter in my chest, so I have to avoid infection and cuts with the vigilance of a long-tailed cat in a room full of rocking chairs.

Cancer is a natural slowing agent, and filmmakers have always understood that it's in slow motion that we learn what's truly important.

In this slow time, I am learning to be patient. I don't try to do several things at once. I concentrate. I do it well (as well as I can, at least), and I do it slowly, whatever "it" is. That slow motion is a reminder to myself that getting well is a life-long process, regardless of how long or how short the life is. The living is in the process, not just in the result. It is important to experience each moment, not just the end.

Take writing this meditation, for example. Dorothy Parker used to say, "I hate writing, but I love having written." I was like that. I rushed through everything I did so I could mark it off the list and go on to the next line. I missed most of my life, because we live mainly in the "writing" and not in the "having written." So, it's tempting to me to get this meditation done, to hurry on to the next one. After all, I have a lot to say, and I don't know how much time I have in which to say it. Isn't that reason enough to rush?

While I'm doing it, couldn't I also pray for those who will read it, and make a mental notation of where I have to be this afternoon while I'm writing and praying? Wouldn't that make the most of my limited time?

Whoa, there . . . Slow down. No one really does three things at once. We just think we do. Actually we switch from task to task with great speed and frequency. But the switching takes time, a nanosecond, regardless of how nimble we are at it. By doing but one thing at a time, concentrating on it, then switching to the next one, we actually save time, as well as wear and tear on our mindbody.

"Having written" is just a small fraction of life. I figure that even if cancer ends my days "early," I'll actually get more living in than I would have with my precancer approach, because I'm experiencing the "writing," too.

Now that I have cancer, I go slow. . . .

. . . I say "I love you."

OH, I've written it on paper once in a while before cancer. I've even said the words occasionally. To the dog when we are out on a walk alone. To my wife when no one else is around. To my daughters on their birthdays. I think I even said it to my parents once. I'm quite open about saying I love the Cincinnati Reds and chocolate mint ice cream and Tony Hillerman novels, although I've never actually said it to a first baseman or a dish of ice cream or my copy of *Talking God*.

I know I scare some folks now. They think I've stopped short of the top floor. "Why does this bald man say he loves me?" they ask themselves. "Rational people just don't run around saying that all the time."

Well, having cancer knocks out a lot of rationality and leaves room for love to move in.

I know saying "I love you" can be very cheap. A movie star goes on a talk show and says to the host she just met, "I love you, daahling." Yes, it's hard to believe it means much. A man says it to a woman in the heat of lust so he can get "satisfied," without giving it much, if any, thought; it's just a means to an end. A child wails it to a parent to escape a spanking. A mother says it to pour guilt on your head at what you have, or haven't, done.

So many folks in our time, however, cannot say it at all. Young couples talk about "the L word"; they can't even speak "Love" out loud, for fear of commitment.

In Charles Schulz's "Peanuts" cartoon strip, Lucy is constantly trying to get Schroeder to fall in love with her.

One day, disgusted with his lack of response, she asked Schroeder if he even knew what love was. He immediately recited the dictionary definition of the word. With a scowl on her face, she said, "On paper, he's great."

We have a lot of paper definitions of love, a lot of songs and poems about it. It's not real, though, until it becomes embodied, in a person.

Helen and I were once in a group of couples. Each person was given pencil and paper and told to write his or her definition of love, without consulting anyone else. Then the leader had each person in turn read out his or her definition. This was a group of highly educated and intelligent people. As they read what they had written, each definition replete with beautiful and esoteric language, my heart began to fall. I could see by Helen's face that she felt the same way. When her turn came, she embarrassedly read out her definition of love: "John, and Mary Beth, and Katie, and Daddy, and Mother, and . . ." She finished, and it was my turn. I read my definition: "Helen, and Mary Beth, and Katie, and Mother and Dad, and Uncle Ted and Aunt Nora . . ."

We sat in silence. Then a strange thing happened. The other persons in the group grabbed new sheets of paper and began to write lists of names!

Love is in relationship, self to self, body to body, spirit to spirit, or it does not exist at all.

I don't know why we have so much trouble saying "I love you," but I know cancer patients can get away with a lot that "normal" people can't, so here's what I propose: Say "I love you" all the time. To everyone—to the man or woman in blue, who's giving you a ticket . . . to the discount store checkout girl who took so long you missed lunch . . .

to the waitress who mixed up your order . . . to your teacher or boss or secretary. Then maybe we can say it also to the folks its really hard to say it to—husband or wife, children, parents, friends.

> *Now that I have cancer, I'd rather take the chance of saying "I love you" once too often than once too little, wouldn't you?*
> *By the way, I love you.*

. . . I don't sweat the small stuff.

I KNOW A WOMAN who has a plaque on the wall behind her desk. In large letters, it says: DON'T SWEAT THE SMALL STUFF! In smaller letters below, it says, "It's all small stuff."

The saying is half-right. The small stuff isn't worth sweating. We spend so much time sweating and fretting and regretting about little things that don't matter. But it's not *all* small stuff. The small stuff is what my colleague and cancer friend, Jean Cramer-Heuerman, calls "ants around the ankles." It seems to me that there's a difference between the ants around the ankles, which aren't worth the sweat, and the details of life, which really are worthy of attention.

One of the things that impresses me most about Jesus is that he paid attention to the details but didn't sweat the small stuff. Remember Jairus's daughter? Everyone thought she was dead forever. Jesus took her by the hand and said, "Little girl, get up." She did, and the entire household was so overwhelmed by joy that they danced and shouted and whooped. They forgot "Tabitha," the little girl. It was Jesus who said, "Look, she's surely hungry by now. Give her something to eat. A piece of fish would be nice."

A piece of fish? What a mundane thing. How could anyone think of a piece of fish when they had just seen someone raised from the dead? How could someone claiming his mission was saving the whole world be concerned with such a little thing? It was a detail, but to the little girl, and to Jesus, it wasn't small stuff.

I think the distinction is this: The details make a difference in people's lives, including my own. Paying attention to the details feeds someone. The small stuff doesn't feed anyone. In fact, it detracts and subtracts from the store of the world's love.

My problem is that so often I get the details and the small stuff mixed up. I can't tell the difference.

I get so worked up about remembering which telephone calls I need to make, and what to say in a particular letter, and whether anyone will get a certain room open in time for a meeting, that those ants around the ankles take over my life. They eat the whole picnic.

Sure, I have an organizational method. I have places I write these things down—many places! I even set my wrist alarm to remind me when it's time to do one of them. The method itself, however, begins to contribute to my sweating of the small stuff.

I become absorbed in how to be ever more efficient. It's like trying not to think of a polar bear. I begin to think about small stuff done and undone as I run, when I pray, as I try to fall asleep at night. The small stuff is like water that seeps into a package of rice; all of a sudden the rice begins to swell and the package breaks.

The world around us doesn't make it easy to give up sweating the small stuff. Many people put a lot of pressure on us to make sure we get small stuff done. One of the reasons the world is in such bad shape is that we spend so much effort on the small stuff. It uses up all our energy. There's none left to put on the details, the details that get people fed.

It's not easy to make the distinction between small stuff and details, between ants and the picnic. For instance, what about doing the dishes? That's one of my jobs. Helen cooks and I clean up. It's a good arrangement, since I have neither the creativity nor patience for cooking. Isn't washing dishes small stuff, though? No, because it makes cooking and eating possible. It becomes small stuff, however, if I spend more than five seconds thinking about it, if I develop a computer program to tell me when and how to wash dishes. One clue that some part of life has become small stuff is when you can't break away from it, when the ants are gnawing at your ankles all the time.

You're sweating the small stuff if you're thinking about it at a time you can't do anything about it. If you're caught in a traffic jam, or waiting for a long train to cross, or imprisoned in a grocery line with a cashier who can't figure out how to scan Spam, there's no point in sweating it. You can't do anything about it! If you're at home, why think about something that needs attention at work? If you're at work, you can't be doing the dishes at home. If there's no solution, there's no problem!

There's so little time, even if I get well and live forty years. There's no time to sweat the small stuff.

The ants are still gnawing, but I'm getting better at ignoring them. That's a gift from cancer.

> *Now that I have cancer,*
> *I don't sweat the small stuff.*

. . . I live in the now.

RIGHT NOW. Today. That's all. Because that's all there is. As one little boy is reported to have said, "There's tomorrow and today, so why can't there be a 'tonow'?"

I feel this, but I'm not sure I can explain it. I'll put it as simply as I can: What "eternity" means is that all of life is telescoped, from the past and the future, into this one present moment.

Looked at from one direction, there is no now at all. As soon as I have typed these words, they are already in the past. The ones that are yet to come are in the future. What we call the present is simply a razor-thin dividing line that keeps past and future apart.

When that divider is removed, however, and past and future run together, there is only now. I think cancer, somehow, removes the dividing line between past and future. When the divider is in place, there is no now at all. When it is gone, there is only now.

I've always been a person who enjoyed both past and future. I like remembering and I like anticipating.

I recall with great pleasure the first time I met my wife. I can even remember what she was wearing. She had on a blouse, or a sweater, and a skirt, and some shoes. The clothes had colors, like green or brown. She also had hair. And she says I never notice anything!

I love remembering how my now-grown daughters looked when they were little girls, and how they used to push me off the sofa when I tried to take a nap after supper!

I recall my grandmother and my first car and going to see the Reds play and marching into Montgomery with Martin Luther King. I like living in the past; it's a good place.

The future is a good place, too. I've had the pleasure of anticipating all those things I've just remembered—our wedding day, and how the little girls would look when they grew up, and a Reds World Series victory. I look forward still—to seeing this book published, and going to support group tonight, and what "heaven" will be like. (I'm not too anxious to find out about the other place!) I like living in the future.

Somehow, though, as I live with cancer, the future and the past are both with me all the time. Remembrance and anticipation are both more real because they are both present, in the eternal now. The division between past and present isn't there anymore. I'm the sum total of everything I've ever been and all that I shall ever be. I used to be a library, full of many books, filled with many stories. Now I'm just one book with one page, but the whole story is right there.

I heard a tale that supposedly took place in the dry section of Nebraska. One farmer asked another why his pigs were so much fatter.

"We pole them," he was told.

"What's that?"

"When it's dry and there's nothing on the ground for them to eat, we tie them to a fifteen-foot pole and hold them up in the oak trees so they can eat the acorns."

"Doesn't that take a lot of time?"

"Hell, time don't mean nothin' to a hog!"

I'm beginning to understand that story, which worries me a little, since it means I'm beginning to think like a hog! Time "don't mean nothin'" because it doesn't exist.

Albert Einstein, when asked to explain his theory of relativity, said, "An hour seems like a minute in the arms of one's beloved. A minute seems like an hour in the chair of one's dentist."

In the arms of God, there is no time. There is only love. That's what we call eternity, not endless time, but endless love. If you have love, you have all the time in the world—right now.

Now that I have cancer, I live in the now.

. . . I'm on vacation.

I T'S A VERY STRANGE VACATION, like none I've ever
experienced before, but still, cancer is a vacation. My
friend and colleague, Jean Cramer-Heuerman, who also
has cancer, understands this. She says we should write essays entitled, "What I did on my cancer vacation." Well,
here's mine. . . .

I'm on vacation from a lot of stuff I used to consider so
important that I just could not get away from it. Commit-
tee meetings. Piles of unread old newspapers and magazines. Unpruned bushes. Unpoisoned dandelions. Courtesy
calls on people I don't like. (A "love" call on someone I
don't like is different.) Getting all my Christmas cards in
the mail on time—whatever "on time" is. Keeping records,
so I'll know tomorrow what I didn't do today, so I can keep
feeling guilty about it. No guilt and no judgment—now
there's a vacation!

I heard about a man who visited from church to church.
He was looking for one where he would fit in. He slipped
into the back pew of a new congregation a little late one
day, after the opening hymn and just in time for the con-
fession. He heard the people intoning, "I have done those
things I ought not to have done, and I have left undone
those things I ought to have done." He breathed a sigh of
relief. "My kind of people at last," he said.

My kind of people, too, until now, when I have cancer. . . .

I'm on vacation from all that guilt. Maybe it will come
back some day, but I hope not. I like the vacation too much.

What is a vacation, anyway? It's a time away from the

regular routine, usually in a different, maybe even exotic, setting. Normal patterns are broken. There's time for doing something we choose rather than things that are required of us. We have a chance to get a different look at the world around us and at the world inside us. Maybe that's why so many people don't enjoy vacations.

When I was "healthy," meaning strong in body and stupid in soul, a vacation always made me anxious to get back to work and routine and anxiety and justifying my existence. I had things to do, battles to win, worth to prove. Now that I have cancer, vacations make me want more vacation.

Don't get me wrong. I'm still working at my job, even during chemo week. Even during "reaction" week, which is worse. The vacation I'm on is a break from judgment, of others and of myself. I just spend my time lying on the beach of love, letting the waters of self-acceptance wash over me.

Come on down. Even if you're on 5-FU, this sun won't burn you, and the water's fine. . . .

Now that I have cancer, I'm on vacation.

. . . I'm getting things done.

T HEY ARE THINGS I'VE WANTED TO DO for years, but I didn't have the time for them. There was no time because I did so much I didn't really want to do. Now I have less time, but I'm doing what I want to do. I'm finally a human being, instead of just a human doing.

I have less time, of course, because of cancer. Getting well is a full-time job, regardless of whether I'm alive or dead, what body I'm in, when the job is done. Surgery, visualization and meditation, chemo and its fatigue—they fill up minutes and hours and days.

I have more time, however, because I have cancer.

First it was recovering from surgery. Most days I just laid on the sofa, thinking and praying. But those were things I wanted to do then. No one expected me to do otherwise. When I had the energy to read, I read what I wanted, not what I had to plow through because of my job.

Then it was the suppression of my immune system by the chemotherapy. I was told to stay away from crowds and public places because I was especially vulnerable to germs and would have a hard time getting rid of them if they got a hold on me. Gradually I began to realize how much extra time I had because I was skipping the expected, whether it was a meeting or a movie.

It's not that I did bad or useless things before. The things other people expected me to do were not unreasonable. No one asked me to murder anybody, except, perhaps, me.

I still take out the garbage and wash the dishes and walk the dog. I still call on shut-ins (if they don't have germs!)

and preach at worship and work at the thousand other tasks that are my job. Someone needs to do those things, and I'm no better than anyone else just because I have cancer.

So what's the difference? If I have less time and more time because of cancer, how am I getting done those things I always wanted to do?

It's a matter of focus, I think. I simply see better what is loving and what is just doing, what is making the time fulfilled and what is just filling up the time. We have this incredible eagle-sized power of love, but we use it to hop around on the ground like one-winged sparrows.

I once lived in a city where I worked downtown. I was walking home after working quite late one night when I noticed that someone had flipped a cigarette butt up onto the canvas awning of a flower shop. It was slowly burning a hole into the fabric. The awning was too high for me to jump up to knock it off. There was no great danger, but I thought the fire could spread and ruin the awning. A phone booth stood on the corner. The fire department was just two blocks down the street. I telephoned the fire house, and explained somewhat embarassedly about the very small nonfire. I thought they might have someone walk down the street with a hand extinguisher.

Nothing happened for a while, and I was just about to walk on. Then suddenly fire sirens split the air! Trucks and cars roared out the big doors of the fire station—ladder trucks and snorkel trucks and an ambulance and even the chief's car! Because of one-way streets they blazed a six-block path through downtown. They arrived at the proper address, and the fire fighters piled out of the trucks. They attached every conceivable hose to all the hydrants they could find. They ran in circles with axes and oxygen tanks.

The only problem was that they couldn't find the con-flagration! By now people who lived in apartments above the buildings were hanging out the windows in their night-clothes. I wasn't about to point out the blaze, thus admit-ting to everyone just who it was who had called this fire-fighting brigade into action!

Finally, in disgust, they began to pack up their equip-ment. Only one hose was left when the last fire fighter saw the "flame." They quickly hauled the hose over to the front of the building, turned on the water, and just blew that whole awning off the building and out into the street!

I think our lives are like that. We have the mighty equip-ment of love. With it we could put out all the fires of hate. We use it, though, on the little charred spots of our daily schedules instead of on the great conflagrations of our daily fears.

Using the time for love, that's the trick. If it's not loving, I just don't do it.

> *Now that I have cancer,*
> *I have time to get the loving things done,*
> *because that's all I do.*

. . . I don't like cartoon shows on TV.

WHILE STILL IN THE HOSPITAL, I started watching cartoon shows on TV in order to laugh. I need to laugh. I want to laugh. Laughter is healthy. When an anvil drops on Wile E. Coyote's head, though, I feel the pain. When Jerry blasts Tom with a cannon, I feel the hole.

So much of laughter is at someone else's expense. We want someone else to pay the price for our fun. We say we "split our sides laughing," but it was because someone else split his pants or head. How often our laughs are based on another's pain or humiliation.

That kind of laughter doesn't do me much good. It is antithetical to love. It is damaging instead of healing. Unfortunately, it's the kind of laughter that is taught to children from the cradle, through the cartoon shows.

Good laughter is a sign of the presence of God. It helps us get well. Bad laughter is a sign of the absence of love. It makes us sick. You see, it's love that heals. Laughter *at* someone else isn't love. It's just meanness. It may even do the laugher more harm than the one laughed at.

One of the most cheerful persons I ever knew was Josephine Petry. Up to the day she died, of cancer, she always had a laugh in her holster, and she was the fastest draw in the county. After I had known Jo for a while, I was amazed to learn of the difficulties of her life. Before we had met her, she had spent six years nursing her husband in illness. In all that time, she never left their home, not once in six years.

I said, "Jo, how in the world could you survive a sentence like that? I know you loved Don and wanted to take care of him, but your home must have been a jail."

She smiled and replied, "Every day I found something beautiful to look at, and something to laugh at."

I have no doubt that in spite of being shut in, Jo never watched the cartoon shows. She was always able to laugh at herself, and, gently, at the foibles of the world.

A certain Roman Catholic cardinal lived a life of devout seriousness. Then he got sick. Everyone, including him, was sure he would die. His relatives came in and started dividing up his belongings. He lay in his sick bed, watching them, angry at their greed and insensitivity, but unable to do anything about it. Then his pet monkey picked up his cardinal's hat, placed it on its own head, and began to admire itself in the mirror. It was so silly that the serious cardinal burst out in laughter, and laughed himself right back into health and life.

That's healthy laughter—a good guffaw at ourselves and our own pretensions and our own failures, not the painful laughter that enjoys another's pain. Laughter is not a sure sign of the presence of either God or love, but God and love use laughter, healthy laughter, to put something beautiful into each day.

I'm much more sensitive to the pain of others now. I can't enjoy another's misery or humiliation or failure. I know what pain and fear are like. I also know how much fun it is truly to laugh with others, to laugh at myself, to laugh for the sheer joy of it.

> *Now that I have cancer,*
> *I don't like, or watch, the cartoon shows,*
> *but I'll be glad to have you laugh at me, with me.*

. . . I clean out drawers . . .

AND FILES . . . AND BOXES . . . and shelves . . . and piles of stuff in the corner . . . and . . .

My first oncologist must be a football referee on his days off. He wanted to tell me how much time I had left in the game. "It'll be over in a year or two."

One of my first thoughts was, "I've got to get rid of my stuff." I have nineteen file drawers of notes and articles and clippings and letters and photographs and ideas. My boards and bricks host a thousand books, or maybe two or three thousand; I lost track a long time ago. I have boxes of old tests from college days and stacks of the high school newspaper I edited. I am surrounded by mountains of important magazines I'm saving to read when I get the time. Strong and hairy moving men have been known to weep upon seeing my "stuff."

Can you sort through and get rid of fifty years of history and another fifty years of hopes in the brief span of one or two rotations of the earth around the sun? I was saving all that for retirement, but . . .

Then I learned from my next, and continuing, physician, Dr. Bernie Siegel, that the football officials might be wrong. What if I don't die in the predicted days? What if I get to write and speak and think and read for another ten or thirty years? Then my drawers and shelves would be empty, and I'd be like Mother Hubbard's poor dog.

If I die unsorted, though, my wife will have to deal with the stuff, which is hardly fair to her. She might not deal fairly with the stuff, either. I mean, she actually likes to clean and put things in order. Our daughters say that on her gravestone, it will read, in Prussian: "She got things done!" The only thing that has protected my stuff so far is that she is afraid of the alien life forms that inhabit my room.

So, a dilemma: to sort or not to sort . . . to toss or not to toss . . . to save or not to save . . .

I have decided the test is usefulness. Can I really use it? Does it have, or can it have, meaning? If it does, I keep it. If it doesn't, I toss it.

It's amazing how much I've dragged around, afraid to get rid of it, when I really had no need for it. It's a good feeling to know that now I have control of the stuff instead of the stuff having control of me.

I've done that with my mind and spirit and body, too— hoarded up so much on the theory that I might need it some day. Then I just got used to having it around, until it clogged up all the space in my mind and spirit and body.

Now that I have cancer,
I'm cleaning out the drawers—of all my rooms.

... I live in the open.

N O, I D O N ' T M E A N I've taken my sleeping bag out under the stars. I'm certainly not out in the backyard barbecuing—have to watch that fat and smoke! I'm just not trying to hide anything anymore.

Of course, in some ways there is nothing I could hide. Once in the hospital a nurse was working on me. My wife stood down at the bottom of the bed, shifting around, trying to shield me from any passersby in the hall. I finally said, "Honey, don't worry about it. There's nothing I've got that everyone in the county hasn't seen by now."

That's not really what's out in the open now, though, especially since I got out of that backless gown. I'm talking about all the things we keep hidden about ourselves because we're afraid they're not acceptable, that people won't like us or respect us or—worst of all—love us, if they know the truth about us.

I've learned from cancer how dangerous secrecy is. Cancer hid itself in the dark places of my self and grew a tumor that I didn't even know was there. It wasn't until I got opened up that we could do something about that tumor.

So it is with the rest of life as well. Things hidden down inside grow and get bigger until they take over life, and threaten it entirely. The phrase for this is "shame." We are so ashamed of something that we keep it locked away, in the dark. Psychologists tell us that the difference between guilt and shame is that in guilt, we think "I did something bad." Guilt can be healthy sometimes, because if we really did do something bad, guilt reminds us to go get forgiveness, to make the bad thing good. Shame, however, means "I *am* something bad." If I am something bad, there is no forgiveness, no way to make the bad good.

There is, of course, a healthy and legitimate sort of privacy. There's no reason to speak out loud every thought we ever had, to tell the story of every thing we ever did. Indeed, there are good reasons not to do so, such as not boring to death everyone around us!

We dare not use the healthy sense of privacy to cover up shame, however. It is appropriate to choose carefully where and when and with whom we are open, but if we are to get well, in the open we must live.

Through the years a number of members of Alcoholics Anonymous have done the fifth of their twelve steps with me. They sit down, sometimes with what looks like reams of notes, and simply pour out all the bad things they ever did, all the ways they hurt people, while under the influence of alcohol. Often they chose me for that role because I was safe. Some of them were people I never saw before or after. They didn't have to face me every day, knowing that I knew. It was good to choose someone like me. It could have been very hurtful had they shared that list of shame with a spouse or friend or co-worker or neighbor. It was necessary and important that they come out into the open with *someone*, though.

Most of us have addictions. They may not be to substances, such as alcohol or drugs or food or chocolate. They may be addictions to activities, such as sex or running. They may be negative activities, like not eating. They may be to thought patterns—negativity, defensiveness, anger, unrealistic optimism, denial. Addictions are based on shame. They live in the dark. They make us sick, mentally and physically.

We need to take that "fifth step," the step of honesty and openness, with someone appropriate. If our hidden places don't manifest themselves as addictions, but we have the uneasy feeling that something is pushed down inside of us, it would be a good idea just to sit down with someone we trust and think that through, do some looking together to be sure no monsters can hide in the dark.

Getting well means getting honest.

Now that I have cancer, I live in the open.

WHEN IT'S TIME FOR NEW WAYS

. . . I don't prepare.

I JUST GO AHEAD AND DO IT, whatever "it" is. I've stopped getting ready, stopped preparing. I figure all that time in my life I've spent getting ready is for what I'm supposed to be now.

If you've already read of my worries about cleaning out my boxes and file cabinets (". . . I clean out drawers," on page 142), you know that I have a fondness for keeping things. I'm not really a collector. It's just that I think this article or that scribbled note might be useful some day. I just want to be prepared.

Helen could easily toss all that stuff in a dumpster if I weren't around to help, but I'm afraid that if everything gets thrown away unsorted, there might be lost a nugget or two that one of my daughters or a friend would like to have. There might even be a forgotten milkbone, since Waggs likes to give them as gifts and also hide them in case the great dog-treat famine comes.

I remember reading a Halford Luccock column about a man who loved macaroons. He hid them all over his study—in books and file folders and piles of unread magazines. He was absentminded, so he promptly forgot where he put them. Then every once in a while, as he worked and rummaged in his piles of things precious enough to save, he would come across a "macaroon unaware." It was a serendipitous treat. I didn't want to die with any macaroons unaware not turned up.

So I started going through my files and piles, things that seemed so important in earlier days. I'm still sorting, because I'm enjoying it, and because I find I can throw things out now that I formerly needed for security, the way Linus clings to his blanket. There are things I have in my mind and heart now, and no longer need to keep in a drawer.

Also, however, there comes a time when you have to stop getting ready and start doing. I've spent my first lifetime getting ready to live. Now, in my second lifetime, my cancer lifetime, I'm doing it.

I was also the type who not only had to keep stuff, but I had to have the proper equipment with me, too. I keep a ball cap and glove in the trunk of my car, just in case I come across a game that needs another player. I keep prayer cards there, too, in case I'm driving by a hospital and remember there's someone there I need to see, and I don't have my briefcase with me. Of course, that never happens, because I *always* have my briefcase. What would I do if I got an idea and had no pen and paper?

Well, what I'm doing now. I'm in the doctor's examining room, waiting for him to work his way down the hall. There are no books or magazines in here—just tongue depressors and cotton balls. Here I am, with this great idea for a meditation about not preparing, and I don't have anything with me on which to write it! So I'm scribbling on the back of a prescription pad with a nurse-chewed pencil stub I found on one of those little tables. It works fine.

I'm not suggesting we should do away with insurance or never carry a comb or hankie. What I'm saying is that I'm learning to trust the Spirit. Like Abraham finding the ram to sacrifice in place of Isaac, what we need will be at hand. It's probably safe to say that what we need isn't what we think we need; what we need is what we have.

I sometimes feel like I lived more in the first month or

five after I learned I had cancer than in all my previous years put together. Those former years were good years, don't get me wrong. I don't regret them. It seems, though, that they were preparation for this time. I'm no longer preparing; the real thing is at hand. The time for storing nuts away for the winter is done; the time for eating them is here.

Now that I have cancer, I don't prepare;
I just live.

. . . I accept gifts.

WHILE I'VE BEEN ON CHEMOTHERAPY, and had the Groshong catheter in my chest, my blood's been so thin I don't dare get a cut; it wouldn't heal. So John Mills cleans out my gutters. Bill Alexander mows my yard. I looked out the window one morning and there were Ross and Paulina Hunt, sitting on our front sidewalk, weeding the flower beds.

I remember one Christmas how Waggs, our dog, got caught up in the gift-giving spree. She went through her collection of bones and carefully left one for each member of the family. Mary Beth, who was a teenager at the time, didn't allow the dog into her room, so Waggs dropped her gift bone for Bethey just over the threshold. She put another in the middle of Katie's rug, one on the couch in my study, and yet another on Helen's side of our bed. It was systematic and thorough; there was no doubt what she was doing.

I'm sure it never occurred to Waggs that she should give anything to us because we had given to her, or that she might get something in return. I doubt that even the smartest of dogs, which Waggs really isn't, can think in such terms. She's never had any trouble asking (begging) for what she wants, without any thought for anything else. Somehow she just wanted to give gifts. It was an act of grace. Maybe that's why *dog* is *God* backward.

I've never been a good taker of gifts. A gift seems to leave the recipient in debt. A little bit of independence is forfeited when you accept a gift. The giver has a hold on you, even if there are no strings attached to it in a literal way. It may be no more than a word or telephone call or note of thanks that is required, but there's always something.

That's why we have so much trouble living by grace, whether it's God's or someone else's. Grace is free, unmerited, no-strings-attached giving. Nothing forfeited to receive. No thanks necessary. It is so hard to believe that there can be a gift, a love, like that.

If we've been lucky, we've had someone in our lives who loved us that way. In the early stages it is often a grandparent. My grandmother never seemed to run my life, but her presence was always a blessing. She loved me and was proud of me and was willing for everyone to know it. I knew she'd love me regardless of what I did. Perhaps that's why I always wanted to do whatever would please her.

There are others who have reached out to me with grace-filled love, but I've never found it easy to take. Now, though, my resistance is down. There is so much I can't do for myself. I don't even have the energy to write thank-you notes. I'm so far in debt that I can never repay what others have done for me. I have to take, just because I need, without hope of "paying back," making the scales even, being sure I never owe anyone anything.

Now that I have cancer, I'm learning not only the meaning but the reality of grace. I can receive a gift as just that, a gift. If cancer can bestow a blessing, then I'm receiving one—the gift of grace.

. . . I don't keep score.

I DON'T COUNT UP how many pages are left to read in
the book. I don't count the seconds in my stretching-out
exercises. I don't count the number of catches when I jug-
gle. I don't figure up my mileage or my speed when I walk.

Love does not keep count. Love trusts the spirit and lis-
tens to the body. Love stays in the moment instead of comparing it to moments past. Love doesn't count on degrees
and statistics and records and personal bests for its justification. Love reads because it's good to read, runs because
it's good to run, stretches because it's good to stretch. Love
does not keep score.

There's something within us that wants to keep score,
that wants the records to prove where we've been and to
point the way to where we might go. Masons have degrees,
soldiers and police have ranks, academics have levels of
professorships, students have grades, organizations have
goals, businesses have sales charts. Baseball statisticians
can tell us how many left-handed batters from Pennsylva-
nia whose names begin with W have hit triples on July
Fourth, and the last time it was done, and the odds of Wal-
ter William Winchell, a "triple" himself, hitting one this
season.

In its own way, cancer is a record-keeping disease. There
are times I have to take Levamisole at home, outside the
watch of the chemo nurses. (Levamisole is a sheep-worm
medicine. I appreciate it because not only is it getting rid of
my cancer, it's also taking care of my lifelong fear of getting
sheep worms!) I have a chart on which I record each Lev-

amisole dose. The nurses also want charts of diarrhea episodes and blood workups. My oncologist has a "protocol" that tells him what to do with me each month. In the early days of chemo, I kept a journal of my side effects— when they came, how severe they were, what happened.

As the chemo routine settled in, however, I began to realize the doctors and nurses weren't paying much attention to the records. They glanced at them and filed them, but then they put the emphasis on me. I wasn't just a history, a bunch of statistics. Once they were satisfied that nothing unusual was going on (as if everything about cancer isn't already "unusual!"), they trusted their instincts, they trusted me, and they trusted the spirit. I stopped keeping my records and started listening to my body. It's a much better guide.

I'm not saying there's no place for history or records or statistics or scores. If you live by the statistics, however, you die by the statistics. Living by the scoreboard means we have no other way of knowing if we're doing okay. Living by the scoreboard indicates a life that has to be justified, a person who feels no right to be here unless she or he can show the world that record of production. That's the kind of person who is most likely to get cancer.

One thing we cancer patients know better than anyone, perhaps, is that you can't live life as a statistic, and that statistics aren't a very reliable guide, either to the past or to the future. Your spiritual chances are much more important than your statistical chances. Keeping faith is more important than keeping score.

In the Rocking Chair Softball League (men over forty), we have a scorekeeper for the games, but she sits up in the stands and drinks Cokes with her friends. We usually don't know what the score is, even who won, until we're through playing, and we're not sure how reliable it is when we hear it. We've learned to play because it's fun to play, not because it's fun to have more runs than the other team. That kind of competition is usually not fun at all; it can be quite deadly.

Some will say, "What's the use of playing if you don't keep score, if you don't know who's ahead, if you don't know who won?" If you can play, you're ahead. If you played, you won. If all you know is the score, then you don't know the score.

Now that I have cancer, I don't keep score.

. . . I'm learning to be silly.

I MAKE UP SILLY SONGS AND SILLY JOKES. I use my time in silly ways, like juggling and working picture puzzles and building model airplanes. My imaging and visualizing and daydreaming are silly. I'm amazed by the world.

I didn't use to be silly. I was responsible. I was efficient. I was productive. I was serious—deadly serious.

What's the difference? Silliness is much more responsible and efficient and productive, that's the difference. Being serious is what's really silly.

I could do serious imaging, about weighty matters, and people I don't like, and injustices that make me angry, and how the world is going to the dogs—if it hasn't already. I know how to do serious thinking about great problems for which I have no solutions.

I used to do that serious kind of visualizing. I imagined what I'd say if someone did something nasty. I argued with imaginary opponents about angry issues. I awfulized the breakdown of the car or the death of a friend. I anticipated getting caught in a traffic jam or in the slow line at the bank. I spent a lot of time being serious. It made me sick. Now, that was really silly!

If we're silly, however, that means we're serious about being healthy. Norman Cousins found that when he laughed at the silliness of the Three Stooges, he began to get well. Serious medical people said that was silly. Wasn't that silly of them?

At the very least, silliness keeps me from thinking depressing thoughts, the sorts of images that lower the numbers of healthy agents in the body. Prayer is the same way. If I'm praying for myself or for others or for the world, even if the prayer is doing nothing else, it's using up my mind and energy so they can't see images and think thoughts that are negative, that will make me sick. Of course, some people think prayer is silly, too. They're right, of course. Prayer is silly, and silliness is prayer—and they're both good for us.

When children begin to have too good a time, adults say, "Now you're acting silly," or "Don't be silly!" I think adults are jealous of children. We aren't allowed to be silly, so we don't want them to be, either. "Get that silliness out of your head, child. Be serious. Be mature. Live a life of drudgery. Show how adult you are by getting sick and dying young."

I read the results of some medical research on two identical hospital wards with identical patients. The patients in one ward recovered better and faster than those in the other. The only variable was that the ward that did better had student nurses and the other one didn't. "Those silly, little student nurses," as one head nurse described them to me. They were silly enough to be enthusiastic, to believe their work made a difference, to trust that their patients really would get better.

Attitude makes a difference. Silliness is the best attitude. You get sick on serious, you get well on silly.

Jesus said, "You can't enter the kingdom of heaven except as a child" (Mark 10:15 and Luke 18:17). How silly. All children do is play. Why does he think we spend our whole lifetimes trying to mature, to stop being like children? Children are silly. They don't understand how serious the business of life is.

Ah, the "business" of life. But life isn't a business, is it? It doesn't have a profit-and-loss sheet, a bottom line.

Life is given to us as a joy. Little children understand that. There's no business to what they do, they just do it. They look in wonder at the world about them and start laughing and roll down the hill.

I'm sure Jesus had childlikeness, not childishness, in mind. Child*ish*ness is when we think of no one but ourselves and our own immediate needs. It's a stage we need to grow out of if we're to live well with other people. Child*like*ness, however, is a stage we need to grow back into as adults, the stage when life is such a wonder and so much fun that we fall down laughing at it.

We want to be childish when we first hear that we have cancer. We're scared and hurt and we can't think very far beyond ourselves. Getting well is moving from that childishness to childlikeness. Cancer helps us to get into heaven, because if we want to get well, we have to become like children again. Indeed, our task as adults, and especially as patients, is to become more perfect children.

It would *really* be silly not to be silly. No one gets well that way. "It's never too late to have a happy childhood."

Now that I have cancer, I'm learning to be silly.

. . . I recycle everything.

I N THE CANCER CENTER where I get my treatments, there is a recycling bin in the lobby. "Why there?" the noncancered visitors wonder. "These people are fighting for their lives," they say. "These cancer patients won't be worried about the rain forests. They aren't concerned about tomorrow, because they might not have one. So why would they even bother to recycle?"

If you are a cancer person, I suspect you know why. Life in the world is too precious to waste. Every can and bottle is valuable, because every tree is important and every foot of land is holy.

Recycling is a symbol that something used, and even used up, can come around again in a new form, to give new life. We understand that.

Recycling is a way of acknowledging the interconnectedness of all life. In that way it is like prayer, which unites us with every creature through the source of love and creativity and constant renewing.

In the huge, extended McFarland-Pond family, until my generation there were only two cases of cancer. Those two were people deep into their eighties. Now, though, in my generation, I was struck by it at fifty-three. As I write this, my brother, only forty-five, has just undergone surgery and is starting chemotherapy and radiation. Why is this? Why does the incidence of cancer keep rising, until one out of every three people in America will hear that word applied to them?

There are many reasons, but one of them is that we've

polluted our water and soil and air and spirit. We live now in a world made unfriendly by our own technology. It is a vivid reminder, however, that the world is one. If there are cancer agents anywhere, physical or spiritual, none of us is safe. None of us can claim family health history or geographical place or status in the economic order as a barrier to cancer. We're in this polluted world together.

Recycling is a symbol of taking responsibility, not just for our own lives, but for the life that we all share. It is also a way of expressing hope in the future.

Besides, we understand recycling because we are trying to do it with our own lives.

I once heard Reuel Howe tell a story from his childhood. He grew up in the Pacific Northwest. His father lost his job and decided to homestead in the great forests. He took his wife and children and what possessions they had and trekked miles down an almost totally overgrown logging road to a rundown, leftover logging shack. Before they had been there one day, the shack caught fire in the early morning hours. Everything they had was destroyed.

Reuel was a teenager. He and his father walked back out of the woods and into town, where they were able to get tents and supplies. It took them all day. When they got back, they found that Reuel's mother had taken the little children and scouted around the site. They had found a rusty old tin can, some wild flowers, and a tree stump. The flowers were in the can. The can was on the stump. They were sitting around it, playing games at their new table, with its magnificent centerpiece.

She had taken a desperate situation and recycled it and made it good.

Now that I have cancer, I recycle everything. I just want to be in the habit. I want to recycle my life the way Reuel Howe's mother took a desperate situation and recycled it. Life and its parts are too precious to waste, even if I won't be a part of it in the days to come.

. . . *I worry about how much my treatment costs.*

NOT JUST WHAT IT COSTS ME AND MY FAMILY DIRECTLY, but our whole insurance group, and the entire health care system. It's easier to see my own costs, though, and to wonder what will happen to us if my insurance runs out. What if we have to take all our savings just to pay the extra expenses, like transportation and meals and sometimes an overnight stay?

They tell us not to worry, that anxiety suppresses the immune system and makes it more difficult to get well, but how do you not worry when the bills mount up, and you wonder whether you can keep on working, or if there will be a job for you when the treatments are over?

I have good insurance, but no insurance policy covers everything. Many patients have poor insurance or none at all. Not many of us have an extra hundred thousand or so buried in a tomato can in the backyard.

What do you do? Buy lottery tickets? Hope Ed McMahon comes through with one of those clearinghouse sweepstakes? Hit up your brother-in-law for a long-term loan?

Am I really worth this kind of money and this kind of worry? Is my life productive enough that everyone else should pay more for insurance because I'm the one who got sick? Should my family sacrifice new coats and vacations and cable TV so we can spend all our extra time and money on the trips to get my treatment and the extra medicines to counteract the effects of the chemotherapy?

Is anyone worth that kind of money? The pope? The

president? Oprah? Geraldo? The director of Mickey Mouse at Disney World? Is there anyone we couldn't get along without, and won't someday have to get along without?

When you look at it that way, I guess I'm as important as anyone else, because I'm no more important than anyone else.

Each of us comes on stage and speaks our piece and goes off again. Some have better lines than others, but none of us built the stage in the first place. Neither did we assemble the audience. We can move the furniture around some, to make a path for the other actors or to make them stumble. We can ad lib or flubb our lines. That, however, is about as far as our power goes. We didn't write the play, and we have no idea how it will end.

It's not how much we produce in this life, how effective and efficient we are, that gives us a reason for being. Production is usually good, but not always. We've spent billions on nuclear and chemical and nerve weapons that are not "good" for anything. Efficiency is often good, but not always. The Nazis were terribly efficient in dealing death. The world would be a far better place if discount-store clerks had been in charge of those concentration camps!

I'm here because I belong here. God put me here. I am a part of creation. If I can "do" some good, "give something back," that's fine and dandy. But that's not why God put me here. God put me here to be a part of creation, not to do something to creation.

No part of the world is here because it is useful. It is here because it is here. That's true for rhinos and spiders and hawks as well as humans. If I say they have a right to be only so long as they don't get in the way of productivity and efficiency, only so long as they are "useful," then I have no

163

complaint when the world wants to do away with me because I'm using rather than useful.

I still worry, but I only have to worry about where the money will come from, not about whether it's all right to spend my share on getting well. I don't mean to oversimplify. I know there are hard choices here, for me and for society. I also know, however, that God has made each of us in creation as important as every other one. We belong here just because we belong to God and to one another.

Now that I have cancer, I belong. I think I have learned that from looking at the world around me.

. . . *I live in my body.*

MANY PEOPLE DON'T. I know, I've usually been one of them. I was formerly a brain that used a body. My body was a handy tool for getting my brain from place to place. I know a deep-muscle therapist who says most of her clients want to drop their bodies off, let her work on them, then come back to pick them up! They don't even want to spend their spare time in their bodies, let alone live in them.

The body, however, is our home. Our bodies are temples, but we usually treat them more like motels. The basic reason disease happens is that we don't live in our bodies. We do things to our bodies that we wouldn't do if we lived there.

I have a friend who says, "If you want to be well, come home. Inhabit your body."

This body home has an extensive communication system. There are many "I"s within me, and they are not just the characters that inhabit my brain. Emotions are not just in the brain, but in the body as well. Every hurt we've ever experienced is stored somewhere in the body. There's a "mind" in every cell. Each cell is a microcosm of the whole. Indeed, Candace Pert, the chief of brain biochemistry at the National Institute for Mental Health, says that "the body is the outward manifestation of the mind."

Whenever one part of the body is abused or neglected, it tells the rest of the body about it, complaining of its treatment. All the other parts get upset, for unlike people, the "I"s of the body never forget that they are related, that they depend upon one another, that if one gets sick they all might die.

Now I talk to my body, and I listen to it. I ask each part how it is doing, whether it has any complaints, if the rest of us can do anything for it. I lay hands on the parts that hurt, because that interconnected healing touch is one of the jobs of the hands. I ask the parts to get along together and work together. It's amazing how well my body responds to being treated like some body!

To get well, we have to stop using our bodies, as though they are tools, and live in them, because they are homes.

I've come home to my body. Before, I always rushed through bathing, dressing, even eating. I always tried to do some useful work with my brain while I was also using my body, whether it was running or sitting or showering. Just doing something because it was necessary for my body never seemed to be adequate. I had to do something "productive" at the same time. I had to be efficient.

Now I don't try to forget about my body. If the body is doing something, I stay with it, go along for the ride, remain in the moment, see whether it likes it. I live in it, even at the times of pain.

The little child I hear in a room down the hall in the cancer center has the right idea. He's crying and screaming, "No shots anymore," over and over. Good for you, little fellow. You're living in that body, and you're letting it tell the world how it feels and what it needs. You'll get well faster. (Your parents and doctor might go crazy faster, too, but that's their problem.) I'm not as good at living in my body yet as you are, but I'm working on it.

Many people are impressed with "out of body" experiences. I am, too, but I'm even more impressed by "in body" experiences. Those are what you have when you live in your body. They help you get well.

Now that I have cancer, I live in my body.

. . . I laugh . . .

A LOT.

Although there have been days of worry and discouragement in my life, when I found it hard even to chuckle, I have always loved humor of any kind. Now, though, I go out looking for laughs with a net.

There are many reasons why we laugh. It's healthy. Norman Cousins tells us to. It's almost impossible not to sometimes.

Why do we laugh, though, when the humor is almost designed to scare us?

The doctor told the cancer patient, "You have six months to live." The patient replied, "But doc, I can't even pay your bill in six months." "In that case," says the doctor, "you have twelve months to live." Now why would we laugh at a joke like that? How can one laugh in the face of death?

Well, what else can you do in the face of death? Kim Wagler was my first oncology nurse. Her youthful energy and upbeat style and infectious laugh were as important to me as what she taught me about dealing with the disease and the chemotherapy. A few months later, she learned she had cancer herself, of the breast. "The gal with the great laugh," as she is known to all, found that "black humor" was very appealing to her in those early days of her diagnosis. She was the one who told me about the soap opera for cancer patients, "The Young and The Breastless." Why would a joke like that make a breast cancer patient laugh?

Well, I think the answer is twofold. For one thing, it's just better than any of the alternatives. If you've only got six months, or twelve if the doctor is greedy, wouldn't you rather spend it with a laugh on your lips and a song in your heart than with a moan on your lips and quicksand in your heart?

Secondly, the serious side of cancer is just so scary. What will happen to us? Will we suffer in some terrible way? Will death be an end to all the good things we love so much? Thinking about those serious issues only makes things worse. The most likely result of worrying about suffering is suffering. Laughter may not keep us from bad things, but "awfulizing" won't keep us from bad things, either.

I have a friend who has been in a serious, responsible, important, seventy-hour-a-week job for several years. Before he took it he was known as one of the most humorous persons around. We have always joked a lot together. I came across a funny magazine article that fit his job exactly, poking gentle fun at it. I sent the article to him, figuring he could use a laugh or two. He returned it with a very serious and somewhat antagonistic note that said, "I'm sending it back so you can give it to someone who might see the humor in it." I worry about him. I pray for him. I try to laugh about things for him, because his job has squeezed out of him the ability to laugh, especially at himself. The inability to laugh is the prelude to illness.

It's well known by now that laughter brings out the best in us, literally. A good belly laugh increases remarkably the levels of all the healing agents in the body. The old adage that "laughter is the best medicine," or at least one of the best, has been scientifically proven.

I couldn't do belly laughs after my belly had been cut open from San Diego to Boston, so I had to make do with smiles and chuckles. Any laugh you can muster, though, especially when the pain is at its worst, is not only a strike in the healing lane but a laugh in the face of the devil.

Allen Klein publishes the *Whole Mirth Catalog*. He became a laughter collector while nursing his wife through her cancer, looking for anything that could bring a smile to her face. He made us laugh for a whole afternoon at an American Cancer Society seminar. I ordered a laughter cassette tape from the catalog. That's all it is—people laughing. When I feel down, I pop it in my boom-box and turn the volume up. People laugh all over the house. Pretty soon, I'm laughing, too. It feels so right.

Did you hear the one about . . .

Now that I have cancer, I laugh . . . a lot.

. . . I wear my best clothes, all the time.

MY NEW "OUT OF AFRICA" HAT. My brown boat
shoes or snowy white Reeboks. My fashionable
madras plaid shirt. My "prestressed" green casual
coat, with the hood and wooden buttons.

This is a giant step for mankind, according to my wife
and daughters. Before cancer I had two methods of choos-
ing what to wear. The first was to take whatever came
up next in the closet, regardless of color, cut, or style. The
other was that if whatever came up next was too new, like
under ten years old, I put it back at the far end of the rack,
to be saved for a special occasion.

Well, the special occasion is here. Today is the most special occasion I can imagine. If I have a tomorrow, that will
be a special occasion, too. There will never be a better time
than right now! So today I'm wearing my new "oatmeal"
pullover. If tomorrow comes, look for that ritzy new cor-
duroy blazer. Look out, world; I live for fashion!

Not really, of course. I live for love. Wearing my best
clothes is just a way of saying that right now is the time for
love. I'm sure my mother loved me when she taught me to
hold my good clothes back until that really special time
came to wear them. After all, when I was growing up, I had
only one "good" shirt, and only one pair of shoes, for all
occasions. It was important to take care of what we had.
Who knew when you would get something new?

These days I know more about my clothes than about
how many days I'll have. Who knows how many times I'll
get to wear my Cincinnati Reds baseball cap? No use wait-

ing for the World Series. I'm a Reds fan today, and I want everyone to know it. I'm a life and love fan today, too, and I want everyone to know that. When you see me coming down the street, I want you to know that to this man, *today* is a special occasion.

One of the most poignant stories out of Vietnam was that the soldiers always ate the peaches from their C rations first, so that if they got killed, they wouldn't have missed the best part of the meal. Perhaps that's where this saying came from: "Life is short, so eat dessert first."

Remember the story Jesus told about the wedding feast? (You can read about it in Matthew 22:13–14.) The king who threw the party discovered a guest who had not bothered to put on his wedding garment. It was an insult to the host, who had the man "thrown into outer darkness." "*This* is the day the Lord has made. Let us rejoice and be glad in it." Let's dress like we're glad. Put on your wedding garment. We're being called to the feast, the feast of the eternal now. There's no point in waiting for a better invitation, a more special occasion. We're invited to the party, right now.

Get out that new dress, sister. Put on that bright tie, brother. This is *the* special occasion. You figure you'll only get to wear it once? All the more special. Whoever gets it next will be pleased to have it, even more because you wore it.

Look for me in the Easter parade. I'll be wearing my "Crocodile Dundee" hat, and a blue and red rugby shirt, and tan pants with cargo pockets, and . . .

> *Now that I have cancer,*
> *I wear my best clothes, all the time.*

. . . *I listen to my body.*

OH, I ALWAYS DID THAT, OF COURSE. We all do, to some extent. Our bodies tell us things we have to listen to. We get tired and must lie down. A leg hurts so badly we limp. A stomach churns up so badly it turns you inside out. The throbbing head, the aching back, the pain in the neck . . . they all cry out for attention. They talk to us, and we are forced to respond.

Our response, however, is often just an attempt to get rid of the pain so we don't have to listen anymore to what that part is saying. We basically want to ignore these bodies, keep them quiet. Like children are so often told, "You are to be seen and not heard."

Now I try to listen, to hear what my body is telling me through its pain, rather than just trying to shut it up. Disease is a message, not just about a pain that needs to be obliterated, but about a life that needs to be healed.

Of course, the body does not want to hurt. It speaks to us through pain so we'll do something about what is causing the pain. I heard of a man whose life was so twisted that his friends said when he died he had to be screwed into the ground. That's an awful epitaph, isn't it? There was a man who didn't listen to his body.

I listen to the messages from my body, but I also listen to the body's witness, the statement the body is making about the nature of life. One witness of the body to life is the interconnectedness of it all.

When our daughters were still in preschool years, I had a household accident. I had my index fingers stuck in the loops of a self-storing window screen, trying to raise it, when the heavy glass storm panel fell so quickly that I couldn't get my fingers out. It came down like a guillotine, smashing the ends of my fingers. The pain was excruciating. I thought of all the cusswords I had ever heard, and none of them were even worth saying; they would have been so inadequate!

My fingers were flat and purple for weeks. I had to hold them straight up, above shoulder level, to ease the pressure on them. The girls sat around, clucking their sympathy, and one of them said, "Daddy *all* broke."

She was right, of course. Although only a tiny fraction of my total body was directly affected, I was *all* broke. My entire body shared in the pain. The whole body had to contribute to the healing. One part cannot be diseased without putting the complete body in harm's way.

Another witness of the body, clearly related to the connected nature of life, is love. Love, peace, and joy are emotions that heal the body. Hate, division, and resentment are emotions that destroy the body. Nature, at its core, is telling us what it wants, what we are made for, by the ways our bodies react. If we were supposed to be hateful grouches, our bodies would thrive on strife. They don't, though, do they? Our bodies get well on love and happiness.

The body's witness, to which I do best when I listen, is that we are made to relate to one another, to be connected, in love.

Some of my best friends, who bear with me through thick and thin (literally!), who will tell me the truth, honestly, are the parts of my body. They tell me, "Hey, you're doing something, or not doing something, that makes us hurt. Let's get this straightened out."

Sometimes, of course, all I can do is apologize. Like when I'm taking chemo, and a whole chorus of voices comes up from my body that says, "What in the hell are you doing?" I explain that this is going to hurt right now, but will make us all better in the long run. They accept that, and say, "Oh, well that's okay then. We're glad to cooperate."

So we talk back and forth, but now that I have cancer I do more listening than I do talking. It's amazing how much you can learn when you listen to your friends!

Now that I have cancer, I listen to my body.

WHEN
IT'S TIME
TO SAY "NO"

. . . I've put my megaphone away.

I'VE PUSHED IT TO THE BACK of the closet, along with my brown and white saddle shoes, and my yellow sweater with the big smiley face on it. Sound familiar? You got it—a cheerleader no more!

A lot of people—friends, family members, folks we work with, just people we meet on the street—expect us to be cheerleaders when we have cancer. They want us to jump up in the air, yell "rah, rah, rah," claiming "Everything is fine and dandily, we are winning, oh, so handily."

Well, I'm more likely to sink into a chair, mutter "raw, raw, raw," and grumble, "I feel like a total wreck, or second opinion, I feel like heck."

There's a "Peanuts" cartoon strip in which Charles Schulz has Linus telling Charlie Brown that he would like to be a prophet when he grows up. "That's nice," says Charlie Brown. "The problem is that prophets almost always turn out to be false prophets." "Maybe I could be a *sincere* false prophet," suggests Linus.

Sincerity! That's the mark of a cheerleader, isn't it? Sincerity alone, however, doesn't cut it. People can be quite sincere about things that are very bad. False prophets can be totally sincere, but they are still false.

Don't get me wrong. Some of my best friends are cheerleaders. Especially now. I need cheerleaders.

I love it when my friends tell me I'm still doing good work. . . . "Two, four, six, eight! Who do we appreciate?"

I feel better immediately when my wife proclaims how much she loves me and how she never felt closer to me. . . .

"He's a wonder! He's a dream! He's the captain of our team!"

I need to have a chemo nurse grab a big flag with my name on it and run three times around the treatment room screaming. . . . "Push 'em back! Push 'em back! Farther! Farther!"

I cherish the hugs and pats and words of encouragement that come from all my cheerleaders. They lift me up on a cloud of love . . . and I can fly!

There are times when I've led the cheers for each of them, and times when I do now . . . but those cheers aren't about me. I need their cheers; they need my cheers. We get into trouble, though, if we expect one person to be the patient and the cheerleader, too. I can't lead the cheers for me.

What's healthful and wholesome for me is to be honest about how I feel, not to put on my yellow cords and white socks and claim everything is okay. It's unfair of anyone to expect dishonesty from me.

Imagine this: A runner comes into the stadium full of people at the end of a marathon. He looks up into the stands and sees thousands of people, all sitting on their hands. They say, "You're okay, aren't you? You're not feeling bad, are you? Please assure us you'll make it to the finish line just fine." But he *doesn't* feel good. It's been a long, hard, grueling race. Nonetheless, the runner waves and shouts and assures them everything is okay . . . and is so out of breath everyone else in the race runs right on past while he drops to his knees.

Or imagine this: A runner comes into the stadium, barely able to keep those legs moving. Suddenly the crowd is on its feet—shouting, screaming, cheering. She's swept up in the adulation. A wave of energy comes down and picks her up and hurls her toward the victory line. She's not even aware of her feet touching the track. She reaches back and finds more breath in those depleted lungs. She knows she's a victor even if she falls on her face.

We can't be the cheerleader and the runner both. We need the cheers, but they must come from others. Our strength has to be put into the race itself.

> *Now that I have cancer,*
> *I'm the runner, not the cheerleader.*
> *That's okay.*

. . . I don't do favors for friends.

WELL, NOT MANY, ANYWAY . . .
Dr. George F. Solomon says there is one simple question you can ask yourself to gauge your chances of long-term survival. "Would you do a favor you didn't really want to do for a friend who asked you to?" If you say "yes," there go your chances. That's because you fit what Dr. Lydia Temoshok calls the "Type C" coping style for cancer patients: compliance, conformity, self-sacrifice, denial of hostility or anger, and nonexpression of emotion. It's a pattern we learn in childhood. It's also a pattern that ought to serve us cancer patients well, it seems to me.

Why are all these doctors telling us we have an attitude problem when we are just trying to be nice? After all, we are supposed to keep an upbeat attitude. What better way to do it than to paint a smile on the old stiff upper lip? Shouldn't we shout a cheery "just fine" whenever anyone asks us how we are, regardless of how bad we feel? We don't want to be a burden to our families and friends. Maybe they won't like us anymore if they have to take our pain seriously.

One man in my community is lifted up by some folks around here as the ideal example of a cancer patient. "Dan just kept working right up to the day he died," they say. "You'd never even know he had cancer." They say that mostly when I take a day off from work. I have considered all this, however, and it occurs to me that Dan, as admirable as he was in many ways, is not a good model for me. Dan's dead.

I certainly understand that we are all going to die some

day. I don't blame Dan for his death. If he wanted to work up to the day he died, that's okay. That was his choice, although I worry about some of the people who loved him. They may have felt neglected and left out by his decision.

I don't want to work up until the day I die, though. I don't want to smile and say everything is fine up until the day I die. I want to *live* up until the day I die! That may include some hours on the job, but for many, it won't.

If saying "no" to doing favors is going to help me live, then I'm going to say "no." If telling people I feel miserable when I feel miserable is going to help me live, they are going to know I feel miserable. If getting mad at the world's injustice is going to help me live, then look for me on the picket lines. If breaking down and crying and telling the people I love how much I care about them is going to make me live, then get out the tissues and hankies. (It's interesting that we call that "breaking down," isn't it?)

I'm not afraid of dying (well, not much), but I don't want to be afraid of living, in all life's fullness, either. Many of us cancer patients are more afraid of living, in a new way that will help us, than we are of dying. We'll just slip away quietly; no one will ever know. . . .

Certainly I haven't stopped doing things for folks. If someone asks me for a favor, and I can do it without detracting from my wellness, I'm glad to do it. It makes me feel good. But that's the trick, isn't it? I do it because I want to, not out of that old feeling of obligation. I'm not going to do any more favors with a smile on my face and a frown in my heart.

Now that I have cancer,
I don't do favors. I only do wellness.

... There's no one "worse off" than I am.

N O, I DON'T BELIEVE THAT, but I say it to remind myself that each of us is unique, that we're not here just for comparison purposes.

People always say that, don't they? "You can always find someone who's worse off than you are." I know that's true. I say it to myself all the time, but I resent it when others say it. They diminish me by treating my pain as insignificant unless it's worse than everyone else's. Is no one worthy of any sympathy unless she or he is the only one who is "worse off" than everyone else in the world?

I sit in the chemo treatment room. To my left is a teen-aged boy, his clinch-jawed mother perched on the edge of a hard plastic chair beside him. They are both "worse off" than I am—he because he's so young, she because her child is ill. I'd much rather deal with my own cancer than know it is growing in one of my children. I sneak furtive glances at their faces, the blankness of his and the lines of hers, and I know that by comparison I am blessed.

Across the room, beside the aquarium, sits an old woman. The tiny orange and blue fish do their best to entertain her, but she doesn't even see them. Her eyes are open, but she's looking inward. Her only hair is a patch of scraggly brown, down low behind the left ear of her bullet head. Her swollen legs end in rundown house slippers. She is "worse off" than I am.

To my right is a pretty young woman, the mother of three. I remember her from the waiting room in earlier visits, before the cancer took her breast. She was wearing a red sweater then. Every man in the room looked at her more than once. Now she wears a loose smock and makes herself small as she hunches down in the chair. I still look at her more than once. She knows it is out of concern for her loss rather than appreciation for her curves, and she both appreciates and resents it. She's "worse off" than I am.

I scan the room. I pray for each of them in turn. I try to speak with my eyes, spirit to spirit, saying, "I've got a little extra strength today; take it, and use it." I do it because I know they're "worse off."

If someone else walked in right now, however, and said to me, "Well, just look around you. You can always find someone worse off than you are," that boy and his mother, and the old woman, and the young mother would all stand up and shout, "Get out of here. He's here for the same reason we all are. Don't reduce any of us by comparing us one to another. Each of us is 'worse off.'"

We need to count our blessings, but not as a cover-up for our real problems or like a game of winners and losers, "My blessing pile is bigger than yours."

We who are being healed of cancer, even though we are not all being cured, know that we belong to one another. We understand one another in a way no one else can understand us.

Love us. Love us all, please. Just don't compare us.

Now that I have cancer,
there's no one "worse off" than I am.

. . . *I* have *cancer.*

THAT'S HARD ENOUGH FOR *ME* to believe and understand. It seems to be even harder for some other people. Not only do I have to deal with my own denial, I have to cope with theirs as well.

I'm very open about having cancer. I talk about it all the time, although I try not to say the same things to the same persons. I'm trying, by being open, to pull the fangs of the beast that feeds on secrecy, that makes us afraid because it's hidden in the dark. I'm doing it both for myself and for others. Others don't always appreciate it, though. One way or another, they make it clear they'd be happier if I'd shut up and act like I just have a sprained toe.

Many people praise the patient who acts like nothing has changed as the ideal. They're saying, "I don't know how to deal with you now that you have cancer, so I want you to play along like you don't have it. Don't bother me with it, and I'll like you and praise you for your attitude."

That's a lot of pressure. Implied is the threat that if we don't go along with their denial of our cancer, they might just deny *us.* They might withdraw entirely, and blame us for the new chasm between us, blame us for getting cancer. Whew!

Some folks actually do pull out. I know a cancer patient whose husband said, "I just can't handle this." He left. *He* couldn't handle it? What about her? It's easy to say she's better off without him, but we need our friends and family so much right now that we usually do what we must in order to hang on to them, even if that means acting like it just ain't so.

I heard of a man who had cancer for ten years and never told anyone in his family. He was a salesman, so he arranged to get chemotherapy treatments out of town while he was on his rounds. Once a year he went to the Mayo Clinic in Minnesota, but he told everyone he was going on a hunting trip. Was he just a private person? Or trying to protect his family? Or was he afraid of how they would react?

What should we do when family members and friends want us to go on like "normal"? Some patients are expected to wear a wig even at home, do the dishes even though they are so nauseated they can barely stand, arrange chemo schedules so they can still take the kids to piano lessons, or stay out of sight if they look sick.

Well, things are *not* the same, and if other people can't handle it, that's their problem! We're not doing such folks any good by accepting their denial, and we certainly aren't doing ourselves any good. I don't have the strength now to deal with other people's expectations. All my energy has to go into getting well, not acting like I'm not sick. I'm not going to die quietly so that after the funeral they can say: "Wasn't he good about it? He never bothered us at all."

Jesus had some similar problems with the Pharisees. John tells us about Jesus healing a man who was born blind. The Pharisees really preferred that the man remain blind. They saw Jesus' healing activity as a judgment upon their unwholesomeness, which, of course, it was.

"Are we also blind?" they asked him. Jesus said to them, "If you were blind, you would have no guilt; but now that you say, 'We see,' your guilt remains" (John 9:40–41).

When we claim to have no illness, we cannot accept healing. When we allow others to push us into denial, we're letting them deny us life in the spirit, and quite possibly life in the body as well. I won't get well, in spirit or body, unless I first admit reality.

> *Now that I have cancer,*
> *I have cancer. There! In your face, Pharisees!*

. . . *Some people won't talk to me.*

THEY DON'T EVEN WANT TO SEE ME, and I'm pretty good-looking, for a beatup old guy! I don't look much different. Hair's a little thinner. Lips get red and puffy after chemo. Eyes get sort of slitty, for the same reason. I've got an abdominal scar from L.A. to N.Y., but no one sees that. They don't see the pretty blue catheter in my chest, either. (My younger daughter, an avid Cincinnati Reds fan, took one look at it and said, "Oh, no; it's Dodger blue!")

They don't want to touch me, either. In the meditation called ". . . It's a touching time" (page 118), I tell of how cancer makes us more touchable to some folks, because of our brokenness. That's not true for others. Are they afraid it's catching? Surely not; most everyone knows better than that these days. But there's something about us cancer persons that makes others afraid. One of the men in my support group told us of a man who actually got up from his booth in a fast-food restaurant and moved to the most remote one he could find when my friend sat down at the next table. It's strange, how cancer makes us more touchable to some and less touchable to others.

These folk are like the three monkeys: See no cancer people; touch no cancer people; especially, talk to no cancer people.

Are they just afraid they'll say the wrong thing, like "You don't look too bad for a corpse"? Maybe; none of us wants to stick that smelly foot in our mouth.

I think, however, it's mostly that I'm a walking (slowly, but still walking) reminder that "it" can happen to anyone.

Even them. Especially them. My very presence is a symbol of vulnerability. It's especially bad for those who knew me "before," because I was always so strong, so healthy. Not a symptom of any kind. Then one day I had "it." If it can happen to me, it really can happen to anyone.

If I try to talk to them of death, even of pain or fear, they brush it off. "Oh, you are going to be fine," they say. If I persist, they don't say anything at all. They are gone as fast as a hamburger in a tiger cage. They cross the street when they see me coming.

I wish they would talk with me. They're missing something special. So am I.

I wonder if Jesus felt that way. When he was tried, and found guilty, and nailed to a cross, all his best friends deserted him. Not only did they not want to talk to him or see him, they didn't even admit they knew him. That must have been very lonely.

So I do for those who won't talk to me what Jesus did on the cross for those who persecuted him. I pray for them. They won't talk to me, so I talk about them behind their backs, to God. God and I have entered into a conspiracy of love. The more those folk refuse to talk, the more we talk about them. We don't try to change them. We just love them. I still wish they would talk. It would be good for them. For me, too. But until they have ears and tongues, they are at least going to have prayers.

Better look back, you silent ones. Those sounds you hear are the wings of prayer. Gotcha!

> *Now that I have cancer,*
> *Some people won't talk to me.*

187

WHEN
IT'S TIME
TO SAY "YES"

... I worry about my wife.

I'M SURE YOU WORRY about those who love you, too. We tell ourselves not to worry, that worry doesn't help anything. We go ahead and worry, anyway. It goes with the territory called "love."

I worry about Helen's health; will concern for me make her sick, too? I worry about her future; what will happen to her if I die, or take too much care, or cost too much money? I worry about her peace of mind; how can she work and take care of me and face loss and still be the sane and wholesome person she's always been?

I think this cancer business is harder on her than it is on me. Sure, she's not the one who got cut open. She's not the one who hugs the porcelain fixture after chemo, or gets her eyes glued shut, or has feet too swollen to walk on. I'm the one who had the operation, who gets the chemo, who lives with the symptoms.

I'm not the only one, however, who has to struggle through all these, day by day. In the way of love, she was cut open by the operation. The symptoms make her sick, too.

It's the difference between being the driver of a car and the front-seat passenger. Before seat belts we called that "the suicide seat." It's still an apt name for the passenger on a cancer trip.

When an accident starts, you don't know how it will finish. The car fishtails on the ice and then begins to spin. You look down the road and see a truck coming. You steer with the spin and look for traction. You don't know if you can keep it in your own lane, but you're doing your best. All that is what's happening on the driver's side.

In the passenger seat, all you know is that something is terribly wrong and you can't do anything about it. There is no steering wheel in your hands, no brake pedal beneath your foot, no gear shift or lights or horn that you can use. You can only pray . . . and trust the driver.

It's the same on a cancer trip. The sudden spin starts, and you don't know how it will end. We patients, though, have the wheel in our hands. We're scared. We're mad at the ice and our own lack of attention. We see the truck coming and we know this could be bad. But we've got the wheel. We're in control as much as anyone can be.

Not so with our passengers. They're praying and hoping . . . and trusting us to do our best. Sure, if the crash comes, we steer it so we're the one who takes the brunt, but they're still in it.

It's a helpless feeling for that passenger. I know Helen loves me enough she would do it for me if she could—suffer the knife and the tubes, take the chemo and the nausea, walk daily with the fear. But it's not in her hands. She can only ride along, and pray, and trust me to steer my best.

How I would like to take the fear and uncertainty from her! I can't. When you're the driver, you can't be the passenger, too. I have to trust her, also, to sit quietly and not distract me, to pray hard, to duck when I need to see out her window. I need her to trust me.

It's not totally in my hands. I didn't put the ice there in the dark. I may not be able to control the spin. Maybe that tanker full of fear will hit us yet. But I'm doing my best, and so is she.

Now that I have cancer, I worry about my wife.

... *I have something to offer.*

SOMETHING TO OFFER TO OTHERS—my diseased self. I know that there is healing in helping.

I always had myself to offer, of course, and often did. It's my profession, so it wasn't difficult. People expected it of me. That is a problem for ministers, however, and also for their church members. How much is the pastor giving of his or her self because the other person really needs it, and how much is given just because it is required by the job description?

A diseased self is a different self to offer. Only another injured self can see the beauty and holiness in a cancerous self. When it is offered, it is just because we share in the "holeness" of life. We need one another to fill the gaps.

Only a couple of months after my surgery and diagnosis, I wrote a little piece for a national church newspaper. They titled it, "Getting Sick Is Part of Life; Getting Well Is My Ministry." In it I spoke of how I was trying to get well in public, as a sharing of self with my congregation, because my ability to minister to them in conventional ways was going to be limited, at least until my twelve months of chemotherapy were done.

I began to get letters and phone calls from people all over the country in response to that article. Almost all came from other patients or from people who have friends or family members suffering from cancer. A man called from Tulsa, Oklahoma. He told me how he had just about decided to give up, but that my article had given him the strength to go on. Another telephoned from a small town in Iowa. He informed me that he'd had cancer for five years and had told no one; I was the first person he had talked to about it. A woman wrote to tell me of the bravery of her friend as she suffered. I think she just wanted to let someone know of the beauty of that struggle, someone she thought would understand it from the inside. Some wrote to ask for prayers, for themselves or for loved ones. Many fellow patients simply wanted to write a word of encouragement.

I correspond and am in telephone contact with a whole host of new friends. We share good news and bad, comfort and fear, with one another. Although each of us must walk our lonesome valley by ourselves, we do it in the spiritual presence of others who are walking their particular valleys with courage and strength. We are better because we are together. We are together because we share the disease.

I feel that I have been ordained twice. The first time was to the ministry of the church, when Bishop Richard Raines and Rev. Ed Boase and Dr. Otis Collier laid their hands upon me. The second time was to the ministry of cancer, when Drs. Frederic Haynes and Robert Arrol and Alan Hatfield, and nurses Kim Wagler and Olivia Parker and Becky Elliott, laid their hands upon me.

If you're reading this, it probably means some physician or nurse has laid hands on you, and ordained you, also, to this cancer ministry.

Now that I have cancer, there is healing in helping.

. . . My right leg is bald.

THAT'S RIGHT, MY LEG! Isn't that a kick? The chemo couldn't get my head, because it's already bald. Most of the men in my family have bald heads and a lot of hair everyplace else. We like it; growing hair is the only way we know to be macho. Now here I am with my hairy chest and my hairy arms and my *one* hairy leg! Thank goodness it's not summer. . . .

I have asked my oncologist and the chemo nurses about it.

"Why would the stuff make only my right leg bald?" I inquire.

They have no idea, so they look at me like it's my fault.

"Have you been exercising *both* your legs when you take your daily walk?"

I'm a pretty good athlete, but even I can't walk a mile on one leg!

Hair is important to us, isn't it? Most of us dread hair loss more than nausea or mouth sores or the other side effects of chemo. Hair loss shows—all the time; the others don't. We make a game of it, or make jokes about it, and wear turbans and wigs and baseball caps. We make the best of it, but we don't like it.

What can you do for a bald leg? Sure, I can keep it covered up, but that's almost unfair. To be really empathetic with my friends in the chemo treatment room, shouldn't I go around in shorts and then wear an ace bandage all up and down my leg? One youngster is bald as a cue ball from his chemo. Last time they were in, his father had shaved his own head, too. They wore matching baseball caps. I liked that. I almost feel guilty when I see someone in a wig. I want to say, "Hey, take a look at my leg. It got me, too," but that would be really weird. . . .

I had hair on my head the first thirty years of my life. It's a shame, because it didn't matter much then. Every man in the world in that era, except violinists, wore a crew cut. Crew cuts took almost no work. You went to the barber once a week to get the hedge clippers run over it to keep it flat, and in the morning you ran a hand over it to be sure it was still there. No mirror time necessary.

About thirty, though, I began to go bald. I knew the crew cut would let the bald spot show through like a spotlight. I decided to grow my hair out. I could then comb it over from the side and cover the bald spot. I knew, however, that everyone would make fun of me if they noticed this.

So I started growing a beard. In those days, you were considered at least a Communist sympathizer if you had a beard. Everyone I knew was so busy criticizing the hair on the bottom of my head they didn't even notice I was also growing it out on top!

There was one other problem, though. Trimming a beard and growing hair out takes time in front of the mirror. I had never seen so much of myself. It was shocking! I didn't like what I saw.

One day my wife was passing by the bathroom doorway as I worked away on my face in front of the mirror.

"You know," I said, "I really am not very good looking."

"That's right," she replied, and I knew immediately I had made my statement in order to get an entirely different reply from her.

"Hey, wait a minute," I called. "You're my wife. You're not supposed to agree with things like that."

She returned to the door and leaned against the jam, her arms folded.

"Well, you're never very good looking when you're only looking at yourself," she said, "but you're very handsome when you're looking at me."

She smiled, and I heard the truth in a way I never had before. You're always at your best when you're concentrating on those you love, and who love you, rather than on yourself.

So what am I going to do about this bald leg? You bet; I'm going to comb the hair over from the left one to cover it, and I'm not going to let Helen see me do it!

Now that I have cancer, my right leg is bald.

. . . I've lost my prejudices.

I WAS NEVER MUCH INCLINED to prejudge people, at least not along traditional lines of color or religion or nationality. I have to admit, however, that I had my reservations about certain other categories of folk—insurance representatives and drug dealers and TV evangelists and telephone solicitors and used-car sellers and appliance repairers. . . . I've also been guilty of that most ironic prejudice, the prejudgment of prejudiced persons!

When cancer comes, though, how can you hang on to prejudices? Cancer is an equal-opportunity disease. It knows no boundaries, not nation or language or race or creed. It strikes a schoolteacher as easily as a mass murderer, a nurse as readily as a hobo, a member of the NAACP as quickly as a knight of the KKK.

One of the best things my mother ever did for me was to insist that each person has to be accepted as an individual, without the cost of the clothes or the color of the skin or the direction of the prayer considered at all. Still, I have had my doubts—about child abusers and hypocrites and falling-down drunks.

Yes, lifestyle makes a difference. So do environmental factors. A smoker is more likely to get lung cancer. A pesticide worker probably takes a higher risk than an accountant. Those aren't the lines over which we usually divide, though, are they? Smokers are both black and white. Pesticide workers are both straight and gay.

One of my friends had to drive thirty miles each week to get her chemotherapy. She is a tall, beautiful woman of great self-composure, at that time in her twenties. Two other women rode with her. One was an elderly, wealthy, patrician lady, a product of the "best" families and schools and beauty salons. The other was a bedraggled, beaten-down woman who looked much older than she was. This unlikely trio went each week to the same hospital for the same treatment, in a VW Beetle yet! As they drove home after their chemo, every few miles one of them would yell "Pit stop." All three would struggle out of the VW to throw up in the ditch along the highway. They took turns holding each other up and passing around the tissues and saying "You look awful," and then laughing like idiots.

I don't think they ever went shopping or dining or to the opera together because of that experience. You don't stop being who you are because you get cancer. More importantly, though, you stop judging who others are.

Isn't it strange, how we divide ourselves one from another, by such superficial categories as the color of our skin and the size of our bank account? Cancer doesn't even look at color or creed or condition. Neither does its treatment. If radiation burns, it will burn the same on Christians and Jews. Chemotherapy nauseates rich and poor alike. Mastectomies leave the chests of black women and white women looking the same.

Now that I have cancer, I just don't have time to judge the lives of others. I'm too busy making sense out of my own. I also know that every other cancer patient is a special sister or brother to me, whether poor or rich, Republican or Democrat, black or white (or red, brown, or yellow), rural or urban, Christian or Jew or secularist. Cancer doesn't have many good faces, but this is one that is almost beautiful. What a relief it is, too. No more energy wasted on judging and prejudging. Just humans together, bound into one cancer-fighting army.

Whoever you are, welcome to the fray.

> *Now that I have cancer,*
> *I can't see your skin or degrees or holy books.*
> *All I see is you. You look good, too!*

. . . My attitude is a gift I can give . . .

TO THOSE WHO LOVE ME and who care about me. It's perhaps the best gift I can give, because I can't guarantee anything else. I can't say for sure that I'll get cured and stay around here to love them, even though I'm working hard at it. But that's the point, isn't it? I'm doing my best to deal with it, regardless of the outcome.

I'm not sure you have to work at getting cured to give the gift of attitude. A time comes for some when no amount of work will reverse the movement toward the body's death. There is still the gift of attitude, however, in how we look at death and separation.

There is a story of a dying historian, in a day when medicine was primitive and most people died at home. His family had gathered around his bed. His breathing seemed to have stopped. They couldn't find a pulse. They weren't sure whether he was alive or dead. "Feel his feet," someone suggested. "No one ever died with warm feet." From the bed came some muttered last words: "Joan of Arc did." What a gift to his family, what a token of remembrance—of humor, of history, of the kind of man he was.

Another gift we can give is letting others share the process of our getting well. I don't mean necessarily the process of getting cured, because that will not happen for everyone. Although not all will be cured, however, all can be healed. I'm talking about our relationships, to others and to the world, about forgiveness, about saying good-bye, about taking care of unfinished business, about living in the moment. Allowing our loved ones and friends just to watch us in the process of getting our lives in order is a gift, a way for them to overhear the truth.

Søren Kierkegaard, the Danish philosopher, tells of how he overheard a conversation in a cemetery. He was on the other side of a hedge from a new grave. He made out two voices beside that mound of earth. From the conversation he learned that one voice belonged to a grandfather and the other to his grandson. The man who was son to one and father to the other lay in the grave. The grandfather explained in simple terms about death and new life and memories and healing, terms he would have been embarrassed to use had he known the great and highly recognizable philosopher was listening to him. Kierkegaard said that in those plain words, he overheard the truth, a truth he would not have gotten had he come at it straight on, asking for it, trying to wring it out of his own experience and study.

The truth is usually heard best if it is overheard. Allowing others to overhear, to look over our shoulders as we go about getting well, is a gift we can give now, even if we can give no other.

Our older daughter, Mary Beth, was in her church one Sunday when a man came in during the sermon. He was wild-eyed and carried a case, somewhat like a violin case. He walked down the middle aisle of the long, Gothic-style cathedral, banging the case on the end of each pew as he went. Mary Beth, being a preacher's daughter, always sits up front. In a big church, that means she sits alone; there's enough room for everyone else in the back. So he was even with the second pew, where she sat, before she saw him.

He stopped at the head of the aisle, turned and looked at everyone with his gleaming eyes. What would he do? Did he have a gun in that case? Would he shoot them all, like madmen do in public places?

The preacher there told me that Mary Beth slipped off her shoes, pulled up her skirt, and got into a low, sprinter's crouch. But then the young man, never revealing what was in the case, walked out again.

I asked Mary Beth about it after I had heard the story from my preacher friend, Paul. "What were you doing?" I said.

"I was getting ready to charge him if he pulled out a gun," she replied.

"Good grief, daughter. You could never have gotten to him before he killed you. You should have hid under the pew."

"Well, I knew that if he had a gun and I charged him, I would die. But I thought that might give Paul and the choir and organist and the others a chance to duck down, to get out the side doors, to run for help. There just wasn't anyone else up there, Daddy. In that place, at that time, I was the one."

When you are the only one, in that place, at that time, you have to take action. In this place, at this time, I'm the only one who can give my loved ones the gift of attitude, the gift of doing my best with what I've got, without denial, to be a healer—for myself and for them.

Now that I have cancer,
even though I can't give many gifts,
my attitude is a gift I can give.

. . . I'm a forgiver.

I 'VE ASKED MYSELF, "Why did I get cancer? Have I had some loss that left a vacuum for the disease to fill? Did I need it for some other reason?"

The answer surprises me. I got it so I could do some forgiving. Not so I could be forgiven, but so I could be a forgiver, of others and of myself. It is so strange, because I did not know there was anyone I needed to forgive.

I have always been a model child. I spent my entire life before cancer trying to make my parents happy, trying to make them proud of me, trying to take care of them. I didn't even know most of the time that that's what I was doing.

I also don't know why I took that as my unconscious goal in life. It was almost arrogance, deciding I was the parent and they were the children. Except I doubt that a child can truly be arrogant. I was just a little kid, after all, when I started acting that way.

Oh, there were some obvious reasons why I took on that role. We were poor, and I just felt bad my parents and brother and sisters had so little. I even left high school early to work in a factory so I could help with family expenses. I got a lot of praise from the extended family for being "a good boy." In the culture in which I grew up, it was expected the oldest son would act that way.

You see, it was such a "right" thing to do. How could it be wrong? How can it be bad for a boy to work hard and make his parents proud and take care of his family?

I had done that for almost forty years, even while marrying and going to school and raising children and pursuing a career, when I got cancer. Then, suddenly, I could no longer fill any of my old roles, with anyone.

About four months after my surgery, when I was well into chemotherapy, my parents had a problem. It was the sort of thing that in the past would have had me on the road in a matter of hours, going a state away to solve it for them, to line up the resources they needed, to take care of them, to be the dutiful son. Now, though, I couldn't. My sisters and brothers were many, many states away; they couldn't step in and fill the gap, either. Mother and Dad were left on their own.

The most amazing thing happened; they handled it! They solved the problem. They did what they needed to do, and they did it well. They continue to do so.

Wow, did I feel stupid. I'd been messing in their lives all those years, trying to make things better for them, and I was actually making them worse. They didn't need me to take care of them; they needed me to back out so they could take care of themselves. I'd been playing good son, and they'd been playing grateful parents, and neither of us knew it was a bad game.

So, I've forgiven them, and me.

"But wait," you say. (At least I hope you say it; the flow of this will be ruined otherwise, so cooperate. . . .) "Why do you need to forgive them, and yourself, for being in the wrong roles all those years, if neither of you is to blame, if you were just trying to do good? Why not just get on with your lives?"

That I don't know, but the cancer is a clue. I'd been for giving all my life, that was my role. Because it was so deeply buried, so ingrained, I couldn't get out of it. It took cancer to knock me off stride, off balance, out of every normality, to make me realize I couldn't go on that way anymore. I had to stop being for giving, and start being forgiving.

I got cancer, you see, so my parents could be set free from their child, and so their child could finally be set free from them. Together, we gave me cancer, in order to cut loose. We didn't have a bad relationship, but we had a wrong relationship. Forgiveness is what puts that which is out of balance into harmony.

Is that really why I got cancer? Isn't it more likely to be fat in my diet, or smoke in the air? I mean, isn't that reaching some? Who knows? What I do know is that the presence of cancer caused a very important thing to happen, for me and for my parents. In that sense, that's why I got cancer, so I could be a forgiver.

I don't expect you to have a similar story to tell at all, but I suspect that cancer is giving you a chance to become a forgiver. Look deep. See what patterns and relationships of your life are no longer possible because of the cancer. Then forgive.

Now that I have cancer, I'm a forgiver.

. . . I understand about "big guys."

I N THOSE LAST WEEKS, Benny always called me "Big Guy," or "The Tall One." I knew he wasn't making fun of me, but it was still hard to understand.

Yes, I *am* a big guy. Six feet and one inch, when I had all my hair. Too many pounds to be called slender anymore. I'm the kind of guy you put at first base when he gets too slow to play anywhere else.

Ben himself, though, was truly a big guy. His curly, steel-gray hair topped out more than six inches above my "neater" hairline. He weighed about two hundred and eighty, and not much of it was fat. In high school football he was all-state. When I hugged him I feared my nose would get a belly-button bruise. He was a giant, so why did he call *me* "Big Guy"?

He was a few years older, but we got sick about the same time. His was heart; mine was cancer. He was given six months. They told me a year or two.

He accepted his diagnosis, but not mine. So, we entered into an unspoken pact. I would get well for both of us. He would die for both of us.

Through my year of treatment he knew my chemotherapy schedule better than I did. He never failed to telephone during my week of nausea or my week of mouth sores. His statement was always, "I just want you to get well."

He defied the odds, and confounded the physicians, as he always did. He lived fifteen months, not six, enough to see me through the chemotherapy and to hear the oncologist say that, at least for now, I was "clean." Then he timed his death so I could have his funeral the day before I left for my "end of chemo" celebration trip.

It was in the last six weeks of our pact that he started calling me "Big Guy" or "The Tall One." My chemotherapy was complete and I could visit him in the cardiac hospice each day. One or the other of his grown sons would always be there—each one taller than I. Strangely, the shortest man in the room was the "Big Guy."

Benny and I always acted in a way that befitted big guys, when others were around. We were a macho pair, swaggering down the hospital halls together, impressing the nurses with our deep voices and amazingly funny stories, talking masculine stuff, like pickup trucks and oil viscosity. When we were alone, however, we talked about our wives and children, and whether our grandchildren would remember us. When we were alone, we held hands. When we were alone, we prayed. When we were alone, we cried. I didn't feel that big.

It was then that I understood. It really *is* lonely at the top, up where yours is the *only* head because you're the biggest guy around. It's hard, always being the biggest. People expect you to *act* head and shoulders above the rest, not just stand that way.

Remember the curse they put on Jesus? "He does all things well" (Mark 7:37). How could anyone live up to an expectation like that? No wonder he got into so much trouble. I remember when I was "a promising young man." It was frightening. No one tells you what the promises are, but everyone expects you to keep them. How much worse to have it said of you, "He does all things well."

Maybe that's why Jesus called Peter "Big Guy." (The more common translation is "rock.") Peter was smaller than Jesus in every way that counted. Some people even think it was a slightly cruel joke, calling Peter "Big Guy." When accusations came in the night, he didn't have the heart of a mouse. Jesus knew what he was getting, though. He had no illusions about Peter. Jesus just needed someone to remind him that he wasn't alone at the top.

Jesus had a pact with Peter, too, just as Benny had with me. Peter would do the getting well, the getting healed, for both, and Jesus would do the dying for both.

People think that big guys (and big gals) get through life without pain or problem, whether the size is physical or financial or spiritual. It's not true. Even the largest of the large, the strongest of the strong, has to have someone else to call "Big Guy." You need someone you can look up to, even if you have to kneel to do it.

Now that I have cancer,
I understand about "Big Guys."

WHEN IT'S TIME TO LOOK INSIDE

. . . I can't decide what to buy.

I S BUYING A NEW BOOK AN ACT OF FAITH or an act of stupidity? Can I get enough good out of a new shirt, or should I just try to wear out the old ones while I can? What about that World War II leather pilot's jacket I've wanted since I was eight years old? I found a great one, just like the originals, and it's "only" $250, the lowest price I've seen.

How in the world, though, can I justify a new shirt or a pilot's jacket if I die before I get much wear out of it? Nobody else in the family wears my size. They'd just be more things for my wife to get rid of. Besides, do I have a right to spend anything at all on myself when so much money is going into my treatments?

Health care costs a bundle. Doctors and hospitals are mostly covered because we have good insurance. There are all kinds of extra costs, however, that go with illness—telephone, special food, mileage and motels and restaurants for out-of-town hospital trips. My salary continues, but who knows about the future?

I'm sick from cancer, and I'm also sick of being practical. I want to buy that book just because I want to read it. I want that shirt because I'm tired of looking at all my old ones. That pilot's jacket means more to me than just keeping warm on a winter day. I want to think I'm special enough to be worth a new shirt or a new book.

How do I make these decisions? How do I make any decisions at all?

This is going to sound simplistic, but we make our decisions through love. The "good" decisions are love in action. The "bad" ones are love gone wrong. All our decisions, even the "bad" ones, are made through love. Love is why we have decisions to make at all.

Think of cancer in that light. Cancer is just growth gone wrong. There's nothing wrong with growth. We automatically think of it as good. There's so much of growth that is right and necessary. We cannot live without growth. When it starts coloring outside the lines, however, when the cells start dividing like they're trying to fight off snakes, tumors result.

A bad decision is love gone wrong. Love makes us want to be in relationship with what is loved, makes us hug and hold and admire. Love also makes us hurt when we can't have what we love, when we can't skip like lambs upon the hills with whatever or whoever makes us joyous.

Growth gone wrong is disease. Love gone wrong is disease. Love gone wrong makes bad decisions, choices that hurt instead of heal.

Cancer decisions are love decisions. Like any other love decision, we may make it poorly. We might make it to protect ourselves from the pain of loss or the agony of closeness, rather than making it to increase joy. Either way, it's a decision because of love.

It's funny how cancer affects love decisions. Some are so clear you can see your face in them. Others are like looking into a puddle where someone's stirred up all the mud with a stick.

The big decisions are the easy ones, aren't they? Do I want to get well? Do I want to live in wholeness? Do I want to be part of the solution instead of part of the problem?

The little decisions, like what to buy—how can we tell

what's a loving choice? I don't know. I do know, however, that each decision is a love decision, and that each of us is loved, including me.

> *Now that I have cancer,*
> *I can't decide what to buy,*
> *but I know that love is a gift.*

. . . I have to remember that I'm not just a disease.

TOO MANY PEOPLE FORGET THAT.

"I may have cancer, but cancer doesn't have me."

When I was in the hospital, recovering from my surgery, I knew I had it made when my wife reported a conversation she overheard at the nurses' desk. They were saying, "The gall bladder in 604 needs some juice, and the amputation in 612 is complaining again, but the congestion case in 630 is beginning to settle down. And, oh, Mr. McFarland is ready for bed, too."

I wasn't just a disease; I was a person! I had a name!

If I am not just a disease, then I am not identified by the disease. Cancer is not my middle, or even first, name. That means that a cure for the disease is not the first priority. The most important thing for my life is healing.

If I am cured of cancer but try to live an unwholesome life, I am not healed, and so I am not me. I am still identified by the disease, either by having it or not having it. Jesus once said, "What does it profit you to gain the whole world if you forfeit your soul?" What value is there in cure if it only leads to a longer meaningless life?

That doesn't mean I ignore or deny the cancer. It's as much a part of me as being male, white, and a Reds fan. I'll always have the fear and challenge of cancer. But that fear and challenge can be what leads to healing.

By healing I mean getting life right, being in right relationship with God and the others in your universe and your own true self. In Larry LaShan's words, you "sing your own song." If that wholeness is there, every moment seems like a sudden eternity rather than a past to regret and a future to fret. Maybe that is what religious folk mean when they talk about "eternal life."

I sometimes say that I have lived more in the few months I've had cancer than I did in all my previous years. That doesn't mean the former years were not good. There was some wonderful loving that went on in those years. But the intensity of healing, in the face of death, has been a great gift. I thank God for my cancer.

Some people, hearing that, will undoubtedly say, "Now that you have cancer, you're crazy!" But some of you will understand . . . now that I have cancer, I am not just a disease, and I am not identified by it. It is just the occasion of learning my real identity.

Now that I have cancer, I'm not a disease.

... I want to forget about cancer!

IT'S EVERYWHERE. I stand in the grocery checkout line, scanning the tabloids. "Miracle Cancer Cure Fails Siamese-Twin Mother From Mars." "Brown Rice Causes Cancer," according to "noted Chinese healer, Toe Foo." I get home and fetch the "regular" newspaper out of the bushes. The front page of the "Living" section is dedicated to "Ten Anti-Cancer Recipes Using Brown Rice." The "Perriwinkle People" cartoon strip features a hairless dog on chemo.

On the way home I pass the Deja View Theater. The marquee proclaims "Cancer Ward Nurses from Hell" and "Losing It All," the touching, romantic story of an oncologist and her older but wealthy patient. Four letters, all addressed to me but each with a different and exotic spelling of my name, tell me I can "lick" cancer in my lifetime if I just make a donation to the Meredith Lovely Cancer Research Foundation. (How does Ms. Lovely, famous actress and accessories activist, know how long my lifetime is, anyway?) *Backwards Trails* magazine tells of "Thirty-three Bed and Breakfast Vacations You Can Take to Avoid Cancer."

I switch on the TV and see a public service announcement from the Nuclear Energy Regulating Down South agency (NERDS), entitled "Carcinogens Can Be Good for You." I give that up and try public radio, where a woman from the Tobacco Research Institute for Profits Entirely (TRIPE) is telling three lung cancer patients that there's no real evidence her product had anything to do with it, and besides, taking risks is the American way, and who are they to deny others a chance at the same experience, anyway?

Someone I met eleven years ago at a party for the neighbor's schnauzer telephones to tell me his Aunt Sonya had cancer and lived a surprisingly long time, although he can't remember if it was weeks or years. I riffle through the mail and find that my book club is featuring the latest by I.M. Wilde, M.D., entitled *Schemo Your Way through Chemo with My New Product, "Dreamo."*

I guess all this stuff about cancer was in the air before I got it, but I can't remember it. Oh, sure, the occasional odd article, a guest once in a while on the Fill with Okra show, but all the time?

"I've got cancer, but cancer doesn't have me." I don't want every picture of my life bordered in black, every line in my story penned by chemo, every note in my song sung by radiation.

I'm a cancer patient, sure, but I'm more than a victim. I'm a real human being, with hopes and fears that have nothing to do with cancer. I worry about my children, the ozone, the economy, whether I can make the car payment. They are the same worries I had B.C., before cancer. I rejoice in a joke, a well-turned phrase, the face of an old friend, a snatch of a "golden oldie" on the radio, the touch of my wife's lips. They are the same joys I had B.C.

I can't forget about cancer entirely, and I don't want to. That would not be healthy. Cancer is part of my life. But it's only my body that has cancer all the time. It's okay for my spirit to be free from it once in a while. Yours, too.

Now that I have cancer,
I want to forget about cancer!

. . . *I'm a person . . .*

NOT JUST A PATIENT.

It's hard to know what to call us, isn't it? Are we victims? Patients? Respondents? Conquerors?

Yes, we're victims. We've been attacked. Bad things are happening to us. Sometimes we certainly feel victimized. But if victim is all we are, then there's no hope for us.

We're patients while we're being treated, but we're not just patients, and sometimes we're not very patient at all! We're not patients all the time; certainly we hope to be past treatment some day.

Bernie Siegel suggests cancer "respondent." That's not bad, but it's not very clear. It doesn't roll off the tongue easily, either.

Conqueror? Well, yes, some of us, at least some of the time, but that's not a word that can be used about us automatically, just because we have cancer. Besides, the Apostle Paul reminds us that the important thing is to be more than conquerors (Romans 8:37).

I prefer to think of myself simply as a person, like every other person, except I happen to have cancer. I'm a cancer person.

Now I know that's not a very good solution to the name problem either. It's certainly not going to catch on and sweep the nation. It has its drawbacks, just like the other names. Perhaps we're not supposed to be able to find an adequate name . . . ah, and perhaps that is the point!

When Moses asked God to tell him a name, one he could take back to the people to convince them he really had met up with the divine and that the commandments had come from God, not just from Moses's own brain, God refused.

"I am who I am," God said. "Tell them that."

God didn't want to be tied down to a single name; that was too limiting.

Names are important. They can hurt or they can heal. That's why minority groups and others marginal to power are especially concerned about what name they are known by, because they are particularly vulnerable to being dismissed through some uncomplimentary name.

My family name is Irish. When the Irish first immigrated to America, they were very poor, and uncultured and uneducated. Because most of the Irish family names began with "Mc," we were dismissed as "micks," as in, "He's only a mick." Saloon and shopkeepers put signs in their windows saying "No dogs or micks allowed." Help-wanted signs often bore the legend, "No Irish need apply." We weren't persons, we were just a name.

An experiment was done with grade school teachers. They were asked to grade essays. Some of the papers bore unusual student names, associated with minority groups. Others had standard American childhood names, like Bobby and Susie. Although they were the same essays, "Bobby" and "Susie" got much better grades than the "irregular" names. The teachers reacted to the names and the qualities they associated with them, not just to the essays.

"I am who I am." Perhaps that's a good enough name for any of us. Descriptive names have some value; it would be difficult to converse without them. Personal names have value, too. They are shorthand versions of our own stories. When I hear "Babe Ruth" or "Abraham Lincoln" or "Elizabeth Taylor," I immediately know the story, the lifeline, to which that name refers. Category names, though, tend to hide our individual narratives, obscure who we are in our glorious uniqueness.

> *Now that I have cancer,*
> *I'm a person, not just a patient.*

. . . I don't get mad when I forget to switch the magnets on the dishwasher.

WELL, NOT AS MUCH, ANYWAY.

There's nothing quite as maddening as getting halfway through unloading the dishwasher only to find that the dishes are dirty. I've put four plates, six glasses, five cups, and eight bowls into the cupboards, and they were dirty!

"I'm innocent," I scream at the dishwasher police. "The clean magnet was on the front. How was I to know?"

Yes, I know I should be able to tell by looking, but my wife rinses everything until it's almost clean before it goes in the dishwasher. So, it's switch the magnet to "dirty" and take everything out of the cupboard and put it back in the dishwasher.

We have two magnets. One is brown and has a picture of a sloppy duck and proclaims "Dirty." The other is green and shows a nice, polite swan. It says "Clean" right across the top. It's simple to keep them properly organized. Just take the "clean" magnet off the front of the machine and stick it onto the side when the last clean dish has been put away. Then take the "dirty" magnet off the side of the machine and move it to the front. Simple, right?

Wrong! For some reason, no one else in the family remembers to do this. I alone take on this arduous task of remembrance and action. I am the best magnet switcher in the family, perhaps in the entire county. I *never* forget!

Except sometimes . . . and there's the problem. It's just awfully hard to be perfect. At anything. I, however, have my whole identity invested in switching those magnets at the proper times.

Those magnets say a great deal about who I am. I am an organized person. I am efficient. I get the most out of my time. I'm busy, so I must be important. The world would have a most difficult time getting along without me. How would the world's magnets get switched, otherwise?

I heard a friend ask a whole group of people what had been their most successful day of work, ever. They named days on which they had accomplished great things—got married, turned out 347 parts on the assembly line, flunked an entire class of students, plowed eighty acres, made $5,000. Then he asked, "What was Jesus' most successful day of work, the day he fed five thousand people, or the day he was crucified?"

You don't have to be a Christian believer to understand that, do you? Those five thousand people went full for one day. But Jesus' crucifixion brought into being a two thousand year church. Some times that looks like a better day of work than it does on others, but you have to admit that Jesus' failure that day, his loss, was powerfully successful.

Being perfect, being successful, even being efficient, isn't all it's cracked up to be. You can get a whole lot done, even be sure the magnets are switched every time, and not have accomplished very much. Maybe the successful day is the one where we just get by—survive the chemo or radiation, show a little kindness to ourselves and those around us, grow a little toward wholeness, live in the present moment, which is the Eternal Now. Perhaps it doesn't matter that much if the magnets don't get switched, if perfection is not achieved.

I suspect the dishes will forgive me. I know God will.

Perhaps I'll even forgive myself, if I have any time left over for it after I get this magnet thing straightened out!

Now that I have cancer,
I've learned to go a little easier on perfection.
I don't get mad when I forget to switch
the magnets . . . well, not as much anyway.

WHEN
YOU WONDER
WHAT IT MEANS

. . . *I'm at war against my self.*

I AM A SCARRED AND SCORCHED BATTLEFIELD. I am also both of the armies that charge from foxhole to trench and back again across that weary field of battle. I am the body that has cancer, and I am the cancer that lives in the body. The cancer is a part of me that has run amok, but it is still a part of me, for all that. In trying to destroy the cancer cells, I am also attempting to destroy a part of me. Some of me has to die if the rest of me is to live. The only way I can be more whole is if I am less whole.

No wonder cancer is the most confusing disease! Cancer is also, I think, the most spiritual of diseases.

Life in the spirit is a constant letting go in order to take hold, a continual giving up in order to take in. The spirit is just like a hand. If it is balled up into a fist, holding tight to what it has, all it is useful for is hitting and hurting. If, however, it is open, whatever it holds is free to go, but also it is ready to receive whatever might be given.

There is a physical part of me, the cancer, that must be killed, cut out, eradicated, that my body might live. So also there is a spiritual part of me that has to be destroyed for my own health and wholeness. Just as with the body, my spirit will be more whole if I am less whole.

This is the great lesson of cancer, the spiritual disease. I'm not just at war with myself in my body, I'm at war with myself in the spirit, too.

I'm not saying there is no "devil," no force of evil that exists outside us. There seems to be pretty good evidence that evil has a life of its own, invading and intruding where it truly is not wanted.

There is evil *within* us as well, however, that which would kill the soul as well as the body. Christians have traditionally called this "original sin." H.L. Mencken, the great American cynic, used to say that original sin was the only Christian doctrine for which there was empirical evidence. I think he was wrong about it being the only one, but he was certainly right about the evidence for it!

We don't want to be battlefields. Of course not! People are not meant to live constantly with tension and confusion. We want to be able to choose sides and cheer for one team or the other.

Mayor LaGuardia of New York founded the famed City Center of Theater and Drama. Someone once asked him why, since he had worked so hard to create the Center, he never went to the ballet there. He said, "I'm a guy who likes to keep score. With the ballet, I never know who's ahead." Yes! We like to keep score. Cancer, however, is more like ballet than basketball. If we have to shoot at both baskets, how can we know if we're winning?

Somehow we have to deal with this contradiction. If we don't acknowledge the inward battle and enter into it, if we try for a separate peace, then we can't get well. We can choose one side or the other and resolve the tension, but we give up a part of our own story when we do.

There's an old tale about a hermit in the mountains who was supposed to be exceptionally wise. Some of the local boys decided to put him to the test. One of them held a small, live bird in his closed hand, then asked the old man if it was alive or dead. If he said it was alive, he would crush it in his fist and show it as dead. If the hermit said it was dead, he would open his hand and let it fly free. Either way they would confound the wise man and prove him stupid. But when they put the question to him, the old man simply replied, "It is as you will."

Am I the cancer or the cancer fighter? I am both. Strange and contradictory as it is, that is my story. It is not something outside myself but a part of me that I must let go in order to live, not just to be cured in the body but to be healed in my self. I accept the battle, and know that its outcome is as I will.

> *Now that I have cancer,*
> *I am at war against my self. I trust that I shall win.*

. . . *I live in the present.*

A FRIEND WHO HAS CANCER was in our bathroom recently. She noticed a book I had left there on my "morning misery" table. Its subtitle is *Getting Back to Normal when You Have Cancer.* She snorted a little as she returned to the living room. "There's no such thing as getting back to normal when you have cancer," she said. "Things are changed forever."

I know what she means. I agree with her. Mostly, I don't want to get back to normal, if normal is the careless way I went through life before cancer. I just took so much for granted. I didn't really enjoy most of my life, even though the ingredients for joy were certainly there.

Don't get me wrong; my life fit me well. It wasn't like a shirt that chafes around the collar. But it was like a check-list on a clipboard; I did something and checked it off and went on to the next thing on the list. College? Check. Marriage? Check. Children? Check. Career? Check. I was mostly focused on the future, on what was coming up next on the list, instead of really experiencing what was happening to me right then.

Senator Green of Rhode Island held a seat in Congress up into his nineties. One night he was at a party when his hostess caught him peering into his date book. "Now Senator Green," she admonished. "Are you already thinking about where you're going next?" "No," he replied, "I'm trying to find out where I am now." Not a bad idea.

Gunther Bornkamm, the Bible scholar, notes that in Jesus' time, all his people were either focused on the past or on the future. There were those, like the Pharisees, who tried so hard to live by the law they had inherited from generations past that they failed to get into the now. Then there were those who looked forward so eagerly to the apocalypse, when God would bring an end to the world and separate the righteous from the unrighteous, that they also failed to live in the now. Jesus' accomplishment, Bornkamm says, was that he made it possible for people to live in the present, without denying the reality and importance of either the past or the future.

I think God has used my cancer in that way, freeing me from fretting the future (worrying about what I'm supposed to do next) and regretting the past (worrying about things I left undone) so that I can live right now. I get more "right now" time in a day than I used to get in a year.

I think that surely this is what is meant by eternal life, not just life that goes on forever and ever, but that quality in which all the future and all the past come together in the present, when all of life is right here, in the "eternal now."

When I was young and working with college students only a few years younger than I, I invited one of my personal heroes, Richard Campbell Raines, to lead a weekend retreat for the students. He did so, but with reluctance. He was seventy at the time and had just retired. He said, "I'm not sure I can relate to the students. I live in the present age, but the present age doesn't live in me."

He was probably the best present I ever gave those students. They were delighted that at seventy he had just learned to water-ski, something he'd always wanted to do and never had time for until he retired. He and his age were present to the students in that weekend, and they loved him for it.

I think I understand, especially now that I am older, what he meant. I sometimes feel alien in this world. My internal gyroscope was crafted in an age when horses pulled plows and it was a big thing to have a radio and men went off to fight a war of righteousness in Europe and Asia. The present age does not live in me.

I do live in the present, though, just as Richard Raines did every day of his life. I think that's why he was a hero to me. His present and his presence were so full because he packed all of his vitality and experience into each moment he lived. We don't have to live in the present age to live in the present moment.

The present. Think of its two meanings together. It is both a gift and the now. There's no other time that you can receive a present except in the present, and the only present that can give true joy is the present. The present is a present from God.

Now that I have cancer,
I am freed to live in that eternal now, the present.

. . . I have hope.

I SUPPOSE IT IS POSSIBLE to have hope without a chronic illness or some similar disaster, but I don't think I ever did before. I had a lot of wishes, but hope didn't even occur to me as something I needed.

The apostle Paul, in his letter to the Romans (5:3–5), says that hope comes as the result of suffering. Not directly, of course. Paul says suffering produces endurance, and endurance produces character and character produces hope. So suffering is strained through endurance and character, kind of like carrots through a colander, to produce hope.

Frankly I'm not sure about endurance and character in my case. It seems to me those need to be chosen to be real. I suspect whatever endurance and character I have developed as a result of my cancer aren't legitimate. They are there because I have no choice. There are plenty of days I'd gladly give up the cancer and go back to being a spineless non-endurer and a weak-kneed character. I endure, and show more character than I really want to, simply because I have to.

Hope, however, is different. If I had to choose between cancer with hope, and no cancer but no hope, I'd take the cancer in order to keep the hope. I don't want to disagree with so eminent an authority as Paul, but I think we can have hope even if there are considerable suspicions about our endurability and our character.

It's extremely difficult to define what I mean by hope. I've cast about looking for the right words, but I find hope is more real as a feeling than as a mental concept. The best I can do is this: Hope is the affirmation of life, not just a fact of existence in this body and in this world, but as a reality that transcends the barriers that our skins and the ozone layer set up. Hope is saying "yes" to the whole of life, even if we can see only parts of it. If life is real, then it is real regardless of the container it's kept in.

It's hard for us to see beyond our present containers—our bodies and our world and our years—because they are all we know. Certainly we cannot prove there is anything else. But hope says life is so real and so important that these temporary limits can't be the final word. Hope doesn't need proof in order to know. Hope, like faith, "has its reasons that reason does not know."

I think what distinguishes hope from wishing is that the real object of hope is wholeness—wholeness in relationship to our own true selves, to other people, to the world around us, and, yes, to God. Indeed, wholeness can be described as simply being in the presence of God, although we might use different words for "God." Wishing is wanting, longing for something to be different, to look out into the yard and see a pony where there was only a bare spot before. Hoping is trusting that the bare spots will be filled, because the one who is in all and through all will see us through it all. Our hope is in the one who knows what we need, regardless of what we wish for.

Perhaps a story will explain this better than theories. Stories usually do.

William and Mary College was damaged and closed during the Civil War. After the war it opened but was closed again for seven years. Despite the fact that there were no students or faculty and that the buildings had fallen into disrepair, the president every morning went out to ring the bell. That's hope.

Now that I have cancer, I have hope.

231

WHEN IT'S TIME TO MOVE TOWARD HEALING

. . . I cry a lot.

I'VE NEVER BEEN MUCH OF A WEEPER. I've certainly felt like letting the tears flow once in a while, but I learned early that tears were not acceptable. Even in the dark of a theater, when the hero's head disappeared in murky water, and only his white hat floated slowly toward the shore, even then I squeezed tight upon my popcorn and my eyelids and told the tears to stay put.

I must have been about seven or eight when I saw *Lassie*, the original film version. I can still remember Lassie leaving bloody footprints on the rocks. I wanted so much to cry openly, to share that noble dog's pain. I didn't, though. I clenched my fists and my eyes and I kept all my sorrow inside. I've wanted to cry for Lassie ever since. Only now, as I write these words, am I able to do so.

I envy women when it comes to crying. My wife and my daughters are good criers. If some scene or action or word reaches in and shakes their hearts, you know it by the streams on their cheeks. They might not believe this, but I've never doubted that tears are good. They know I'm uncomfortable with crying, so they try not to overdo it in my presence. I've always known they cried behind my back, though, and I've always wished I could slip in a few tears behind my back, too.

Now that I have cancer, it seems like I have permission to cry. Oh, I still prefer not to do it in public. I'm not sure folks would understand. They might think I lost my marbles or stepped on a tack. I'm talking about permission to myself, permission to cry when I feel like it.

Sure, some of my weeping is because of anesthesia hangover. Maybe chemotherapy has a tear side-effect, even. I am sure, however, that I weep now because everything is so beautiful.

I walk my dog down beside St. John's church, the one that looks like it belongs in a German village. I peer up at its tower and stained glass, through my chemo-stuck eyelids, and I cry. I see a finch at the thistle feeder or a squirrel scampering up the TV antenna, and I cry. I examine the face of my wife or see a friend coming toward me or watch Barry Larkin run down a sure hit and throw the runner out, and I cry.

When I cry, it seems like everything is in balance, in right relationship with all other things, that I'm right at the heart of Love. So much is wondrously beautiful. I can't even begin to tell about it. No words are adequate. So I have to cry.

I know there are tears of sadness and bitterness and grief, but I'm not sure they are very different from the tears of beauty. We cry only because of love—because of its absence or its presence. In that way, tears are the sure sign of the reality of love.

I came home one evening when our daughters were teenagers to find them rocking back and forth on the living-room sofa, arms locked around each other, weeping as if their hearts were truly broken. Gently I tried to get my arms around them and whispered, "What's wrong? Why are you crying?"

Katie looked at me over Mary Beth's shoulder, with streaming eyes, and choked out, "I don't know. She hasn't told me yet."

We don't really have to know why another is crying in order to share the love and beauty, do we? Tears unite us in the ways of love and take us into the depth of beauty.

Now that I have cancer,
I cry a lot—and when I cry, I know everything is okay.

235

. . . *I say good-bye.*

I DROVE THROUGH HOOPESTON, Illinois, where we once lived, and I realized I might never see those tree-lined streets again. They hold good memories for me. Our daughters were teenagers then; they learned to drive on those streets. Our older daughter, Mary Beth, graduated from the big, yellow-brick high school there. We loved walking down those streets on a Friday after supper, the four of us under a canopy of old and sheltering trees, to the welcoming little library, where we would check out our "weekend books." The people who live in the houses that line those flat, prairie streets were very kind to us, especially during the several months when Helen's mother was dying.

As I drove over the massaging bricks and attention-grabbing potholes, I understood that I might never be in Hoopeston again, except in my mind. I needed to say good-bye to those streets, although not to their memories.

So I said, "Good-bye, Hoopeston. I'm glad you were a part of my life, and I thank you for those good years you gave us. I may see you again, perhaps many times; who knows? But if I don't, that's okay. I hold you in my heart. Please remember me in yours."

Helen and I walked together on the winding paths of the Indiana University campus in Bloomington. IU is where we met and married. We made friends there who remain close and dear to us. I recall those gentle hills and limestone buildings with great affection. Dogwood and redbud trees in bloom always make me want to study for exams! My college years opened to me doors of scholarship and friend-ship and love that I did not even know existed.

As we left, I said, "Good-bye, IU. I love you still, but I know I may never see you again. I hope that's not true, be-cause I would like to return to this wonderful well to slake my thirst many times. But if I don't, if this is the last time for us to be together, that's okay."

I'm not quite sure why I need to say these tentative farewells to the places of my past. I'm not even sure I need to be there in person to wave that fond good-bye. Perhaps doing it in my mind would be enough.

I do know that commitment to life as unfinished business is one of the marks of a long-term survivor. Saying these in-terim farewells is, I think, a piece of unfinished business.

When I was told I would be dead "in a year or two," my first thought was, "I can't even use up my return-address la-bels in a year or two." Think of that: They are not useful to anyone but me, and to me only if I'm alive. I figured one of my main tasks of unfinished business would be to use up those labels. The problem is that every organization in the world that wants money from me, and there is no organi-zation in the world that doesn't, keeps sending me more return-address labels as a little gift to try to shame me into shelling out some bucks. My unfinished business will take two hundred years at this rate!

Occasionally someone says, "What do you think the best age for a child is? Infant? Three? Wouldn't you like to have them cute like that again for just a day?" We always say, "No, the age they are right now is the best age, because it's the one they're supposed to be."

Life is always a process of letting go of what has been so we can take hold of what will be. That doesn't mean we forget the past. Even old folks whose minds have left them keep in their bones and tissues the remembrance of all the places they have been. We cannot live in the past, however. God is always moving us forward.

Cancer is a forceful reminder of that truth, and I am thankful for the reminder. So I say my tentative farewells. Each one reminds me that I live in an "in-between" time. "In-between" is not a bad place to be.

Now that I have cancer, I say good-bye.

manent limp, but he got a blessing from that encounter. The limp was a reminder of the blessing. Every step he took, Jacob knew he wasn't a "normal" man. You can't wrestle with an angel, even the angel of death, without knowing you have been changed forever. Jacob had his limp. I have my semi-colon. Some have a lopsided bosom or a lonely kidney. For some the mark on the body is gone completely, but the shape of the angel remains on the soul.

I may never "have" cancer again, but I'll never be free of it. It's my companion forever. There will always be the worry, and there will always be the blessing.

> *Now that I have cancer,*
> *I am a captive of the morning.*
> *It's morning when the day begins.*

. . . I want to pretend that everything is still the same.

I'M RECOVERING FROM AN OPERATION, that's all. Nothing is different. I don't need to prioritize my time, or conserve my strength, or meditate, or read wellness books, or go to support group. Everything is going to go back to the way it was. The more I act "natural," the sooner my life will be back to normal, I tell myself.

I know it's not true, though. Life will never be the same for me again. I might live a normal life span, whatever that is, but I'll still have to take the tests and watch for the symptoms.

Being a cancer person is like being an alcoholic. Even if you've been "dry" for five years, or ten or twenty, you're still an alcoholic. You can't take that first drink, regardless of how small. You start every meeting by saying, "I'm an alcoholic."

We might get past the stage of being a cancer patient, being treated, perhaps even being tested, but I suspect we never stop being a cancer person. There's always a piece of the mind that remembers, and wonders.

More importantly, we are changed by the experience, whether we want to be or not, and probably even if we can't tell the difference.

One piece of conventional wisdom observes that as we age we become more like ourselves. Cancer is an interruption of that process of becoming more like ourselves, an opportunity to go in some other direction if we wish. What happens in our bodies with the onset of cancer may

242

be out of our control, but what happens in our hearts is not.

So, even though I want to act like nothing has changed, it has. Now I'm faced with deciding what the change will be. Will I become more open, more spiritual, more loving? Or will I be a denier, and let my denial eat at my spirit in the same way the cancer has eaten at my body—secret, steady, eroding.

I once heard someone say that life is far too much trouble unless you can live it for something big. I would add that cancer is far too much trouble unless you can use it for a change in the direction you need to go.

Maybe it's a change you've always wanted to make and just never had the energy or the courage. Perhaps it's a change that is only now occurring as a possibility. It may even be a change that is forced upon you by the circumstances. Whatever, it's your cancer, so it's your change.

I heard about a frog who was hopping down a dirt road. There were two long ruts in the road, worn there by big trucks that occasionally had to use the road. As he hopped along, he spied a friend sitting down at the bottom of one of the ruts.

"What are you doing down there?" he asked. "That could be dangerous."

"Yes, I know," sighed his friend, "but I fell in here by accident, and I've tried and tried to jump out, but I'm just too tired. It's impossible for me to get out."

The first frog went down to the pond to get some help, only to see his little frog friend arriving minutes later. What a surprise.

"What happened?" he asked. "I thought you weren't able to get out of that rut by yourself."

"Well," replied his friend, "a truck came along in that rut, and I had to get out."

> *Now that I have cancer,*
> *I want to pretend that everything is the same . . .*
> *but it's not. That is, at least potentially,*
> *cancer's gift, to get me out of my rut.*

. . . I believe in miracles.

LEE ATWATER was a "mean" guitarist and a mean campaign manager for George Bush. He believed in destroying the political opposition in any way possible—not just in beating them, but in obliterating them. He took great pride in being nasty. He was only forty when he died of a malignant brain tumor. Before his death, he wrote these words:

> I acquired more wealth, power, and prestige than most.
> But you can acquire all you want and still feel empty. . . .
> It took a deadly illness to put me eye to eye with that truth,
> but it is a truth that the country, caught up in its ruthless
> ambitions and moral decay, can learn on my dime.
> I don't know who will lead us through the nineties,
> but they must be made to speak to this spiritual
> vacuum at the heart of American society, this
> tumor of the soul.

Lee Atwater died, yes. There was no cure for his body, but there was healing for his spirit. The tumor got his brain, but not his soul. His conversion to peace from power, to love from greed, to hope from cynicism, was a greater miracle than a thousand cures. The miracle is always in the healing. If the healing also brings about cure, let us rejoice and be glad. The miracle, however, is in the love.

That's a good definition of miracle, I think: It is the appearance of love where unlove ruled before. Miracle is marked not so much by some otherwise-inexplicable phenomenon, but by the presence of God. Love, which is the presence of God, is what makes a miracle.

Miracle occurs wherever the *attitude* of triumph, the attitude of love, appears, not any actual event of victory. Miracle is not about living or dying, but about getting whole. Lee Atwater is a miracle.

Sometimes the wholeness of miracle, of love, occurs in the body, sometimes in the spirit, sometimes in both. It is not the cure, however, but the wholeness that writes *miracle* across our lives.

A Roman Catholic priest tells this story of his cancer. I first heard it twenty years ago. I understand it now in a way I couldn't then.

He began to feel weak and went into the hospital for tests. There he first heard that word. The tests showed he had cancer.

He said, "I walked out with no anger, no discontent. It seemed that a great calmness came over me."

The hospital said there was nothing that could be done for him, no treatment, but that when he got bad enough, they could send him to Houston where he could be put into an experimental program. He accepted the diagnosis and waited to get worse.

His weakness continued. He could no longer do his regular work. He was able, however, to say mass occasionally for a group of cloistered nuns, those who do not leave the convent at all but spend all their time in prayer. One of the nuns there, Sister Catherine, told him that she would spend full time praying for him until he was well. He just smiled; it was a nice gesture.

Finally the cancer had advanced to the point that he could go to the experimental program in Houston. He looked forward to it. By being a guinea pig, he might at least help the researchers learn something that would help other patients. They ran him through all their tests. Then the head researcher called him in.

"Father, why are you here?" he asked.

"Why, because I've got cancer, and they told me when I got bad enough . . ."

The researcher cut him off, with a wave of his test papers. "You don't have cancer, Father, anywhere. We've run every test in the world on you, and you have no cancer at all."

The priest walked out of another hospital, on another street, with the same feeling of great calmness that he had felt before, the same calmness both upon hearing he had cancer and upon hearing it had left as mysteriously as it had arrived.

"It was then," he said, "that I realized that in the calendar of saints, it was Saint Catherine's day."

That is a miracle story in several ways, but I am impressed more by the miracle of healing than the miracle of cure. Please don't misunderstand. I love cures. I want to be cured. I want you to be cured. The final cure, though, is death. Each of us will die some day, of something. The miracle I see in this story is that calmness of spirit—in diagnosis and weakness, in cure and strength—the same awareness of the presence of God, of the presence of Love.

Now that I have cancer, I believe in miracles.

. . . I steal donkeys.

I T'S PALM SUNDAY, so I want you to go into town and
steal me a donkey," Jesus told his disciples. "If anybody
catches you, tell them I need it."

Reminds me of the time "Gunner Bob" Reinhart, one of
my classmates, happened to notice the keys dangling from
the ignition in Mr. Bothwell's new Olds Rocket 88. It was
Sunday afternoon, and Gunner decided to take the car for
a spin. Mr. Bothwell saw his own car taking off from in
front of his house and ran down his driveway after it, house
slippers on feet and Sunday funnies in hand.

"Why are you taking my car?" he cried.

Gunner yelled back, "I need it."

You can imagine how much ice that cut with Mr.
Bothwell.

One of Jesus' disciples nudged the other as they walked
into town, and said, "If they go for that, I've got some nice
recreational lots along the Dead Sea I can sell them."

All sorts of economists claim Jesus, but he didn't belong
to any of them. His approach wasn't economic at all. He
just borrowed everything. He borrowed the water he turned
into wine, and the stone jars from which that wine was
poured. He borrowed a boat from which to teach or by
which to cross a lake. He borrowed houses in which to eat,
teach, and heal. (Some of them did not fare very well, either—one lost its roof so a paralytic could be lowered in to
be healed.) He borrowed sons and daughters, brothers and
sisters, husbands and wives, to be his disciples. He borrowed the upper room in which he ate his last supper with

his borrowed friends. Borrowed was the manger in which he was born, borrowed his cross, and borrowed his tomb.

Jesus is extolled as a giver, not a taker. He was the giver of health, love, truth, and even the ultimate, his own life. Yet Jesus throughout his entire career "borrowed" things.

This was not just his lifestyle as an itinerant rabbi and philosopher. He was teaching us that all we have is borrowed. He ignored all strictures against lending and borrowing, be it a cloak or a second mile or even one's other cheek, because none of us really has any possessions. Bigger barns, Swiss bank accounts, even gaining the whole world—none of that is enough for us to establish a claim upon ourselves. You yourself, your very life, is borrowed from God, so how can you claim anything you have as you own?

That's why Christians call Jesus "the Word of God." We say he's God's message, God's way of teaching us, God's "mouthpiece," if you will. Not just by his words but by his life, he taught us that we do not belong to ourselves, but to God.

Gunner and I learned in Sunday School the accounting theory of faith. You get what you have coming to you. Indeed, Gunner got it when he returned Mr. Bothwell's car. One doesn't steal donkeys—or Oldsmobiles—and get away with it in my hometown.

Jesus taught the grace theory, that we are borrowers, that we have no claim upon life or God except the one that is given freely, without strings, in love. Grace has no contract requirements, nor can it be attained through manipulation. Grace is what we borrow, knowing we can never repay, and knowing that Love the Lender understands that we can never repay.

We cancer patients work at getting well, and so we should. We take chemo and radiation. We visualize and meditate and laugh. That work isn't very useful or effective, however, unless we understand that even it is a gift. The only reason we try to get well is because life is worth living, and the only thing that makes life worth living is love. Why should we get rid of cancer in order to live a life of unlove? But love is always a gift, always borrowed, always grace. By my work I might be able to get you to respect me or fear me or appreciate me or honor me, but there's nothing I can do to get you to love me. Love comes wrapped up, as a present, as something we borrow for a while from the great storehouse of Love.

The God of Love comes to us and says, "Borrow from me. Borrow the things that make for life. Let others borrow as well, and do not hinder them. Hell is a life that is earned. Heaven is a life that is borrowed. Borrowed is best. Go steal me a donkey . . ."

Now that I have cancer, I steal donkeys.

. . . I am broken.

NOT JUST BROKEN INTO PIECES, although that is true in part. Nor am I only broken in spirit, although there's some truth there, too. My confidence in my own invincibility is certainly broken. I just never got sick before. Cancer struck other people, not me. There's hardly ever been any cancer in my whole large extended family. Now that confidence, that pride, that arrogance in my own healthiness is broken.

That's not all bad. The Psalmist says, "A broken and a contrite heart, O Lord, you will not despise" (Psalm 51:17). For you see, God uses broken things. That's not all God uses, but God does use broken things.

God uses broken things to create learning. Tommy Lasorda's son died at the age of thirty-three. The longtime Dodger manager said, "If the good Lord had come to me and said, 'I'll give you a son, but you can only have him for thirty-three years, and then your heart will be broken because you'll have to give him back,' I would still have held out my arms and said, 'Hand him over.'"

God uses broken things to create sharing. Jesus broke the bread in order to share it at his last supper, and it could not be shared until it was broken. Reuel Howe tells about a dancing teacher who was paralyzed and in a wheelchair. "I could not teach," she said, "until I was paralyzed. Always before I was so involved in my own dancing I was unable to share it with anyone else. Now that my body is broken, I can share my dancing."

God uses broken things to create power. Think of the

atom. It is simply a tiny particle, until it is split. Then, what power! That is in the very nature of things, the way God has made the world. The power follows the brokenness.

God uses broken things to create healing. That is seen most easily in the work of an orthopedic surgeon, who often has to break a bone so that it can be reset to heal properly. We cancer patients understand this. We often have to be broken quite literally, have a part of us broken off—a breast or colon or kidney—so that we can be healed.

Oscar Thomas Olson once told this story. As a boy he begged and pleaded for an air rifle, until his father finally bought one for him. One day he was up in the barn loft, shooting his new gun, when he heard the breaking of glass. He remembered that the old-fashioned storm windows from their house—the wooden-sash type that are removed in the spring and reinstalled in the fall—were stored in the loft. Sure enough, there they were, piled together in a vertical stack against the wall. The pellet from the air rifle had broken the panes in every window except the last one. Quickly young Oscar Thomas moved the unbroken window to the front of the stack, to hide the evidence.

His summer was ruined. He got no joy from his new air rifle. Every day brought him closer to autumn and the day the windows would be brought out to be installed on the house. To make matters worse, his father seemed to go out of his way to brag on him, to tell all their friends and neighbors and relatives what a good boy his son was and how proud he was of him.

Finally the boy could stand it no longer. He went to his father and told him how he had broken all the windows.

"Oh, I knew that," said his father. "I was just waiting for you to tell me."

"I never felt so close to my father in my whole life as I did right then," Olson said.

God uses broken things to bring us back and to bring us close—broken bread, broken relationships, broken bodies.

Now that I have cancer,
I am broken . . . and that's okay.

WHEN
YOU'RE
LOOKING
BACK AND
FORWARD

. . . I want to fail my tests.

OR A CANCER PATIENT, negative is positive. The best news we can get is that there's nothing there. Our top grade is a zero.

I suppose cancer patients are the only people in the world who always want to fail their tests. It's the one time "negative" is a good word for us.

"What did my tests show, doc?"

"Nothing."

Now there's a good conversation!

It reminds me of the time Yogi Berra was hit on the head by a fly ball. They took him to the hospital for X rays. This was the report: "They X rayed Yogi's head and found nothing." That's funny, of course, especially because it was the strangely philosophical Yogi, but it's also good news. There is often a significant "something" in the reality of nothingness.

I worry about that nothingness now, because I'm no longer on chemo. The things I'm doing to try to stay well are not medical. There is a comfort in chemotherapy or radiation. Even the side effects we so much dread are signs that we are doing something to chase down those speedy little devils. As long as we're *doing* something, we have some control.

One of my friends lost her beautiful, long, red hair during chemo. With treatment over, her hair began to grow back. She said, however, "It's almost frightening. My baldness was a sign I was actively fighting the cancer. Now I can't help but wonder if anything else is growing back along with my hair."

So we go to our tests with a little bit of fear. What if I don't fail this time? What if there is something instead of nothing?

I don't think there's any way to overcome that fear. We meditate and pray and love and stay busy, but there will always be a little bit of brain that is wondering about those tests.

Perhaps healing is always in absence, in nothingness. Peace of mind, wholeness, happiness . . . all these depend on being free, of getting to zero. As long as we're lugging a lot of baggage around we're not free. If we depend upon the "things" of our lives to give us meaning, we're not yet whole.

That's the exact opposite of how we usually define success, isn't it? Success is getting more, not getting rid of what we've already got. "The one with the most stuff wins." Whether it's money or cars or promotions or victories or sexual partners, the one with the most is the "successful" one.

Cancer teaches a different lesson about success. The one with the least is the victor.

What did Jesus say? "Go, sell all that you have, and give it to the poor. Then come follow me." It's like the potlatches of some early Native Americans. Instead of having battles where they hit one another with tomahawks and took the "spoils" of war, they had battles of giving. The tribe that was able to give more was the victor. What a highly civilized way of waging war—and we call them "savage" and "primitive."

It's not just because we've been able to get rid of all our cancer cells that we're victorious. The "successful" one is the one who fails the hostility test, too, and the nastiness test and the prejudice test and the unkindness test and the . . .

I think about Jesus, on his way to Jerusalem, knowing what faced him there. He had to fail his test, too, you know. Think of all the power he had, enough just in the fringe of his robe that it could heal, enough in his vocal cords that he could call Lazarus out of the grave, enough in the soles of his feet that he could walk on water. His test was to *not* use that power, to become a nothing, to stand silent before his accusers, to say, "*Not* what I will . . ."

He failed his test. Such a failure is called "salvation."

We cancer patients understand that. If we fail our tests, that's good. We know, though, there will come a time when we must fail like Jesus, when we must give up the control, give up the power of chemotherapy and radiation, when the body will give up its very existence. That's good, too, because it is part of God's plan to lead us on, to places where these bodies cannot go.

Now that I have cancer, I want to fail my tests.

Bibliography

Here is a listing of books mentioned in the meditations.

Anderson, Greg. *The Cancer Conqueror*. Kansas City: Andrews and McMeel, 1988.

Borysenko, Joan. *Minding the Body, Mending the Mind*. New York: Bantam, 1988.

———. *Guilt is the Teacher, Love is the Lesson*. New York: Warner Books, 1990.

Cousins, Norman. *Head First: The Biology of Hope*. New York: E.P. Dutton, 1989.

Dooley, Tom. *The Night They Burned the Mountain*. New York: Farrar, Straus, & Cudahy, 1960.

Hill, Albert F., with Paul K. Hamilton and Lynn Ringer. *I'm a Patient, Too*. New York: Nick Lyons Books, 1986.

Klein, Allen. *The Whole Mirth Catalog*. San Francisco: Allen Klein.

Ryan, Regina Sara. *The Fine Art of Recuperation: A Guide to Surviving and Thriving after Illness, Accident, or Surgery*. Los Angeles: Jeremy P. Tarcher, Inc., 1989.

Shideler, Mary McDermott. *In Search of the Spirit*. New York: Ballantine Books, 1985.

Siegel, Bernie S. *Love, Medicine, & Miracles*. New York: Harper & Row, 1986.

Siegel, Bernie S. *Peace, Love, & Healing*. New York: Harper & Row, 1989.